Being There

Being There

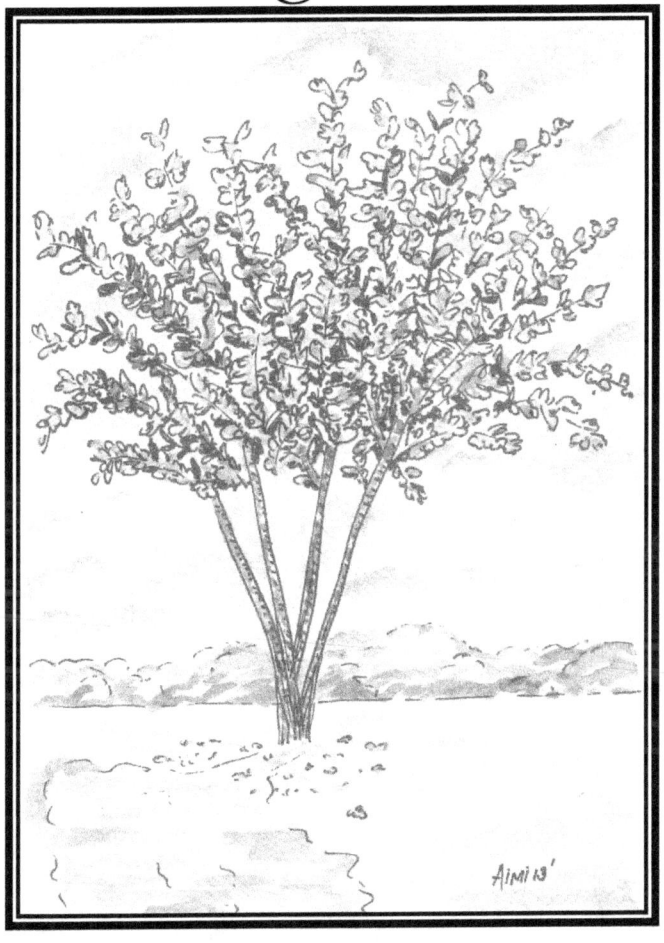

A daughter's voice for her father's silence.

Aimi Medina

CONTENTS

DEDICATION

I dedicate this book to my father. He has had to stay silent this entire journey. My heart has spoken out for him through my words and tears. I want to thank you, Dad, for giving me the strength to write your story. Your story has allowed me to grow, understand, and appreciate something so difficult and yet so beautiful - we call *life*. I'll always be your baby.

ACKNOWLEDGMENTS

I am grateful to the individuals at the nursing home who were able to patiently find a way to communicate with my dad and allow him to keep his dignity. I want to thank my mom for having the strength to lead us down this most difficult path. I want to thank my siblings Robin, Lori and Darrow for coming together and supporting Mom the whole way there. I want to thank my family, my husband Dave and my two brave children Drew and Jonny, for always understanding. Lastly, I want to thank my dog, Flounder, for his late night snuggles that helped me make it through many sleepless nights. I love you all.

INTRODUCTION

I am the baby of the family. I grew up always trying to keep up with my brother Darrow and two sisters, Lori and Robin. Both my parents, my dad (Leonard) and my mom (Susannah) worked as speech/language pathologists. They worked primarily with elderly stroke patients.

We were a middle class family who spent our summers enjoying the Florida beaches and taking trips to the dreaded mosquito infested Everglades. We didn't appreciate the Everglades much when we were young but Mom and Dad did. Dad loved nature and capturing the beauty of the birds and alligators in his photographs.

Growing up, Mom always took the lead to get us involved in sports and activities. Dad was mostly on the sidelines taking pictures and enjoying us from afar. We knew he loved us all but he couldn't handle us for long periods of time. Things had to be done on his terms. For instance, at dinner Dad would watch the evening news and we could only talk during the commercials. He'd always share his bagels but we knew to never eat the last one. When he had enough of us, he'd retreat to the living room and shut the door. Dad had a temper which was sometimes unpredictable, not just around us but with Mom as well. We didn't understand it but we learned to try to not set him off. That's just the way it was in order for us all to live together under the same roof. We didn't know any differently, so that was normal to us.

As we grew older, both Mom and Dad instilled good moral values in us. They financed our college, had us find jobs to support ourselves along the way, and taught us to save money. They also kept us active and healthy through exercise. Each of us grew up to become the successful adults they'd hoped we'd be.

In his retirement years, Dad loved being a grandfather. He enjoyed being a part of the grandchildren's special occasions. He captured many joyful moments in photos as he did with his own children.

Although Dad was difficult at times, he had a sensitive heart and only wanted the best for us. It's easy to find faults in a person but he did a lot of things right. He raised a family that stood by and loved him to the very end.

Chapter 1

THE DAY EVERYTHING CHANGED

I realized being of the artsy mind, that I needed a way to express and relieve the buildup of this ongoing tragedy. The only thing I could find were my words. Let it out and let the heaviness lay on the paper, not on my heart. And so, I'll let the words paint a picture.

Tuesday, January 3rd 2012

I received a frantic call at work. It was Mom. The dreadful call no one ever wants to get. I could only hear broken words and the helplessness in her voice. "They're taking him to the medical center. He can't move or speak." I let Mom know I'd be there. Little did I know how that would happen. I'm a teacher and it's not easy to leave a room full of children. As my family was my first priority, I made it happen. That's when things became real. That's when I knew things just weren't going to be the same.

Friday, February 17th 2012

Looking back, it was my father's face but I couldn't tell how much of him was truly still there. Hidden behind a massive stroke was the one thing he needed most right now, his words. Little did I realize at the time that it erased so much more. Taken from him was his mobility, written and spoken language and the utmost loss - memory. However, there was one thing it didn't take away. He never forgot who I was. That was reassuring but also painful. It's hard to grasp the concept of how important someone is to you yet not be able to retrieve a life of memories with them. It's just heartbreaking. That's what daily life is like now. It's a realization of the next stage of my life, of Dad's life, of all my family's life. The parents who supported and raised me, now need me the most. It's the most fulfilling thing I can do for them but it's ultimately going to be the hardest.

For you to understand what follows, this journal entry was written on Sunday, June 16th 2013.

After Dad's initial stroke which paralyzed him on his right side, we were faced with a decision that to this day carries such guilt. We were told that a tube through the nose could only be placed in a person for a short time. This tube was necessary as Dad had lost his ability to swallow. They informed us that the doctor was in the hospital at the time and could put in a feeding tube right away rather than waiting until after the weekend. We thought it was the right thing to do. We thought it was the only thing we could do. We had no idea at the time how this decision would change Dad's life and ours. It had been about three days since Dad had anything to eat. This decision is what kept Dad alive. This is where we unknowingly intervened with nature taking its course. In the back of our minds we thought this feeding tube was temporary and would be taken out when Dad learned to eat again. That never happened and no medical professional ever supported us to do so. We all wish now that he could have died naturally, in the hands of God.

Monday, February 18th 2012

I was now taking daily trips to the rehabilitation center where he was first sent for his therapy after his discharge from the hospital. The first visits were tearful. I realized, when I left my father and sat in my car and cried, that it wasn't only for my father any more. It was for all the patients who I'd become accustomed to saying hello to each day. I wasn't just praying for my family to get through this. I was praying for people whose names were not even known to me. This experience was much greater than I could have ever imagined. Each time I walked through those double doors, I knew I was doing the hardest thing possible - being there.

After a number of days, Dad had to move to a more permanent facility. He was entitled to 120 days of intense therapy in hopes of regaining whatever speech and motor skills that were lost. They told us the first six months were critical for recovery. Whatever the patient is able to regain during that time is probably the most they will. The place the rehabilitation center recommended was just across the street. It was a therapeutic treatment residence. I remember the day he was admitted. The head administrator met us at the door. She was boisterous as she strutted around in her high heels and form-fitted clothing. The first thing she blared out in Dad's presence was, "Does he have a living will?" I should have known then that this was going to be a difficult stay for Dad.

My husband Dave, and our sons, Drew 14 and Jonny 12, came to visit Dad one afternoon. This was the first time they'd seen Dad since his stroke. It was quite shocking for them and emotionally overwhelming for Dad. I'm glad they came. It's been hard this last month-and-a-half to explain to my family the pain and disbelief I've felt since this happened. Even more difficult was trying to explain to them just how much Dad had lost. Even though Dad couldn't express himself with words, I knew from his eyes that he missed them all so much and how proud he was of them. It was difficult to watch my kids being so brave and my dad wearing his heart on his sleeve.

Sunday, February 19th 2012

I went to visit Dad today. Mom was on her way to meet me there with their dog, Skippy. Skippy is a white Maltese who used to belong to my brother Darrow. A few years ago, Darrow and his family had to move to Tokyo for business and left the dog with Mom and Dad. They became very fond of this dog, especially Dad. Bringing Skippy along on visits was a reminder of home.

While I sat outside with Dad, he was trying to tell the nurse something. We couldn't figure it out. It's like a game of charades and we always lose. While we tried to decipher what Dad was trying to tell us, I noticed a patient in a wheelchair was being strolled through the courtyard by her family. She looked like she was the grandmother that once held her family together. It seemed like everyone came to see her after church. They were all doting over her. With a few simple words, they were able to understand that she needed to use a bathroom and also was having some back pain. They were able to quickly flag down a nurse and get her needs met. It helped me understand Dad's frustration. He has so many needs and it's as though no one hears him, no one responds and no one understands. It was 11:30 a.m. and he hadn't taken his medicine. I tried to assist the nurses' failed attempts to give it to him. He was demanding. He only wanted to take one pill and not the other that was needed for anxiety and depression. We were getting nowhere. So by lunch time, when Mom and Skippy arrived, he was in complete shambles. He was having an emotional breakdown. Finally, with much coaxing, we managed to get him to take his medicine. What an awful feeling. I felt like a "drug pusher" trying to persuade my father to take medicine that he knows affects him in a way he doesn't like. Yet, it's the only way for him to gain control over his emotions. What an awful road he's on. The worst part is knowing that he took it for me because I told him so. The guilt is unbearable.

Monday, February 20th 2012

I didn't see Dad today. Mom had to bear the task alone. I made my 4 p.m. phone call to her to find out how things went. I make this call every afternoon if I don't see her. She lives alone now so I find it necessary to check in with her every day. I have to take a deep breath before doing so. I never assume things are okay. Happily, Dad took his meds in the morning as scheduled. All went well. It's scary to think that a good day means nothing tragic happened.

Wednesday, February 23rd 2012

As usual I took a deep breath and called Mom for my 4 p.m. update. According to Mom, Dad was in a "psychotic spin" this afternoon with lots of ranting, finger pointing, and swatting at her with his good arm. Mom was coping the best she could. She finally got him from the patio into the building. Then she went out and sat in her car. Sometimes that's the only place she can cry freely and regain her composure for yet another round.

After my phone conversation with Mom, I decided to stop by to see Dad. On the way, I had picked up Drew from school. When we got there, Mom had already gone home. Dad was happy to see us even if it was for a little while. He has lost his short term memory so he probably didn't even remember what went on earlier that day. In his twisted speech, he would vent a little then break into a "half" smile as he gazed peacefully at Drew and me. At least we were able to bring him just a little happiness that day. That's all I could do. I just wish I could bring some to Mom.

That evening my oldest sister, Robin, called. She lives in Georgia with her husband, David, and their two grown children, Justine and Davy. She updated me on the outcome of Mom's current stress test. They planned to do a cardiac catheterization to find out if she needed a stent in her left descending artery. Mom doesn't like me to worry more than I have to so, sometimes, I have to piece the story together by what she tells each of us children. Now it makes sense why she has been so persistent about getting all her documents in order. She wanted to be sure someone would have durable power of attorney. She doesn't want to undergo this medical procedure without having that in place. More importantly, she doesn't want us to deal with similar circumstances if something were to happen to her.

This situation has brought to light the importance of having more than a well thought-out living will in place. Dad had a living will but it wasn't written with the intention of surviving a stroke as severe as his. He checked off three things in his will: a terminal condition, an end stage condition, or a vegetative state. If he became incapacitated due to any of those conditions, it was his desire that his dying should not be artificially prolonged. These conditions are open to interpretation by the medical community. A stroke can be an end-stage condition but medical doctors give a patient six months to see what capabilities they are able to regain. Most people don't improve their physical or mental functions after that point. Dad did not specify in his will which life sustaining treatments he would or would not accept. His will left many questions unanswered. It wasn't enough.

Dad needed a durable power of attorney. A durable power of attorney would have enabled Mom to manage his financial affairs easily and act in his behalf even with him being incapacitated. In his will, he did appointed Mom as his health care surrogate in the event that he became incapacitated. That was a good decision but he needed to do more. Mom was only authorized to make health care decisions in his best interest. She wasn't allowed to take care of his financial obligations freely. She would need to be his legal guardian to do this. I still can't grasp Dad's way of thinking. I look back and think that maybe he was in such denial that he could ever be in this situation - where someone else would have to make decisions regarding his health and be in charge of his money. Now Mom is paying the price for that. She will have to be appointed as his legal guardian and to do that is costly and invasive. A judge would have to determine if Dad is incapacitated. In order to prove that, physicians, psychiatrists, and all sorts of therapists have to evaluate him. They also watch carefully how moneys are spent. Everything has to be justified and documented under the supervision of the probate court. There will be no Medicaid to help. Mom will have to get an elder-care attorney to help her along and protect any assets. We will have to spend all of Dad's life savings and risk there not being anything left for Mom before any government assistance besides Medicare is offered. It's frustrating to think that much of this grief we're experiencing could have been avoided.

Through all this, Dave has been supportive and comforting. He wanted to help in some way but didn't know how. He's a "fix-it" type of person. What he did do was necessary and important. This experience is a lesson my entire family learned from. He took the initiative for us both to sit down and write our own living will. We also appointed each other as durable power of attorney. After doing much research and having all the correct documents in place, he sent copies of the forms to all our family so they could easily get theirs done if needed. There is a whole business side to this tragedy that I didn't expect. I pray Mom has the strength to get through this. Her need for guardianship has been a real headache.

On a positive note, I've been told that Dad is making progress with his therapies. He's walking with a four prong walker and getting a little movement in his right arm and leg. Although I'm glad to see signs of progress, his mental state worries me constantly. Mom talks about bringing Dad home. I just don't know how we could make that work. It feels like an unsolvable math problem. I can't seem to find a formula that can work.

That's what my brain is doing when I can't sleep at 3 a.m. in the morning. I never was very good at math.

Sunday, February 26th 2012

I went to visit Dad for lunch. Mom needed a well-deserved day off. For the past week, Dad has been resistant to Mom and showing disinterest in her visits with bouts of anger toward her. His mental state is now regressing. If we could only understand him, it would be much easier to accept his decline. It would allow for a clearer picture into his true understanding or misunderstanding of the world around him. I often listen to his new language, picking up a word he's recently heard, and listening to him use it over and over. He uses the same word and changes the rhythm and tone of it. He tries so hard for it to have the consistency and intonation of a true sentence. This is something many of us take for granted. So I let him vent to me in his own language while we sat on the patio. He is so sincere about his thoughts, yet the uncontrollable need to repeat the same words over and over again, saddens the truth of it. I can't imagine the world he is living in. I feel such anger that he somehow blames Mom for his condition. Yet I know delusions are a part of this new term being used for these recent behaviors - psychotic.

Blaming Dad, or anyone at this point, for the situation Mom and the rest of us are in requires too much useless energy. It's such a wasted effort and only eats away at you. I think blame is used as a distraction rather than dealing with reality.

Mom is still determined to bring Dad home when the time comes. Even if it doesn't happen, you have to have hope. Whether hope means that he'll be at peace here on earth or up above. These times require so much strength. Sometimes hope is all you have. It is your strength.

Monday, February 27th 2012

I had a nice visit with Dad today. The definition of "nice" has changed since his stroke. Nice means no drastic episodes, surprises, or me breaking down during my visit. Crying after is considered "normal."

I brought Dad a picture dictionary and a dry erase board. I attached letters and numbers to Velcro so he could easily use it if he chooses to. I was putting these together at work before I left for the day. It was a terrible feeling to have to look around my classroom for materials to loan to Dad to help him communicate. A coworker saw me assembling things and made the comment, "Are your students really that low?"(I teach 4th grade.) I took a deep breath, looked up, and told her it was for my dad. Funny, how my project for Dad turned into a lesson for someone else.

Thursday, March 1st 2012

Mom got the paperwork started for her guardianship over Dad. I plan to take the mandatory class with her so that in the event that anything happens to Mom, I will be able to take over. Lucky me.

Mom is waiting for the doctor's office to call to schedule an appointment for her stent procedure. It may be next week due to the push to have it done before they could possibly send Dad home.

According to Mom, Dad wasn't as stand-offish today. I gave her some suggestions on how to deal with him. Rather than telling Dad what tasks need to be done, she should only suggest it. He owns such little independence as it is. So today she mentioned to him to brush his hair. He did brush his hair, but with a toothbrush. We all need to accept that there is a new understanding for "mission accomplished."

Saturday, March 3rd 2012

I took my family to Mom's house today. After Dad's stroke, Mom went into independent mode and has been trying to keep up the house and yard herself. Now, after some time, she's more at ease in allowing us to come up and help her. Dave helped with weed whacking, Jonny got to drive the rider mower, and Drew got to take Dad's convertible for a spin around the block to keep the battery charged. I think Mom's beginning to realize that she can't do this alone. Thank goodness!

Later that evening, I went to visit Dad. He was doing okay. The last two visits, he's been studying the picture dictionary I gave him. Each page has a different theme: winter, zoo, a restaurant, etc. I wonder if looking at the pictures helps to trigger memories of events from his past. I sure hope so.

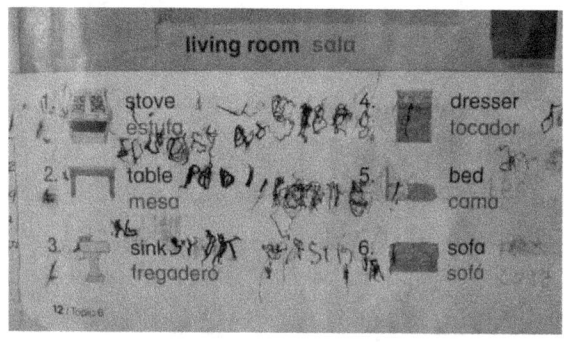

A page from Dad's picture dictionary with his writing.

While there, I met Dad's roommate, George. He explained how he ended up here. He and his wife were visiting from out of town and staying with friends. He had a stroke his second day there. His wife had to find a permanent place to stay as he was too sick to fly back home. They've been here ever since. George's stroke affected the left side of his body. He still can communicate, read, and is very sharp in his conversations. He asked if Dad had regained any feeling from his paralysis. I told him "very little." He said he's talked with many stroke patients and many agree that with the recovery of feeling, comes intense pain which he's experienced himself. I was sorry to hear that. What a lousy tradeoff.

Monday, March 5th 2012

Mom's afternoon update revolved around Dad not eating. He wouldn't even go in the dining room today. They will start giving him more supplemental protein shakes through his feeding tube. Being a typical rotten Monday experience for Mom, she asked if I'd pick him up a greasy burger. I was tired from work, but this was an emergency meal in our family. I'm not sure why I had such a strong feeling to rush there. If he wasn't going to eat the food they served him, then he probably wouldn't eat what I brought. Never-the-less, I picked up a Happy Meal at Burger King. Surprisingly, I made it there before dinner was even served. I felt guilty bringing in fast food for all the other residents to smell but Dad wasn't eating and my focus was on him. With great surprise, he ate the entire burger except the bread. The smile on one side of his face and the "mm, mmm's" were all worth it. Before leaving, I told Dad, "You're the best part of my day" and he was.

Thursday, March 8th 2012

Robin came down from Georgia to help during Mom's heart procedure. We went with Mom to her out-patient appointment this morning. It ended up with the best scenario. They did exploratory surgery and nothing else. They didn't find anything wrong. What a relief. They said the chest pains she's been having must be due to stress and anxiety which is understandable.

Robin and I checked on Dad at lunch time. We brought him a hamburger again in hopes to entice his appetite. We were told that a nasty stomach flu was circulating through the building so they had the patients eat in their own room. Dad ate a decent lunch (for him), so I hope he can bypass this next curse. As we sat on the patio, a man walked by with his dog. It looked like "Mickey" the dog Dad used to have. It struck him hard. You could see his emotion of a dog surely missed.

Monday, March 12th 2012

Robin stayed with Mom for about a week. She was very helpful and supportive with the many issues Mom has had to deal with lately. To name a few, there was the heart procedure, guardianship, a letter from the IRS about Dad's filing, fixing Darrow's car (because she ran over a landscape timber) and Dad. He's always on the list.

We all went to visit Dad on the weekend and had a nice visit. Dad was civil and seemed to be glad we were all there. It's been just over two months since Dad had his stroke. I've grown-up so much in such a short time - not by choice but by circumstance.

Dave has been transferring our old movies to DVD's these past two weeks. On the TV, we watched the years pass quickly in front of us. It's been quite an awakening. I've accepted that my children are teenagers. I can now appreciate their childhood rather than feel depressed that those baby years are over. I've also watched my dad in the videos as I mostly remember him. I can watch them now without crying and appreciate those times we had. I can accept the person he was and move toward accepting the person he is today. He's still my dad - plain and simple.

Monday, March 19th 2012

Okay, it's official. Mondays are bad. The pattern I'm seeing here is one step forward, two steps back. Mom visited Dad today. She said he was acting out and resisting coming back into the building. This is the second time in two visits that she's had to seek help to bring him back in. Due to this regression, the home visit to assess the house for his homecoming has now been canceled. He's the main roadblock at the moment. I can't express how frustrating it is to watch Mom struggle so hard to get him home and he can't grasp the big picture. He probably never will. As I researched his condition, it's looking more and more like senile dementia on top of the severe stroke. It's awful that I'm jealous of many of the other residents who are there. Now that's pathetic! It seems to me that most of the other patients have the ability to clearly communicate their wants and needs. I see how easily we can take speech and emotional stability for granted. The facility is already suggesting that home health care may not be enough for Dad. I know Mom will sacrifice everything of herself for him to come home. My hope balloon is deflated today. Hopefully, it will be full again tomorrow.

Tuesday, March 20th 2012

I visited Dad today after work. Mom took the day off - well understood. The therapists caught me on my way in so I went in to talk with them. They updated me that Dad is plateauing and has been resisting therapies. They plan to discharge him next Wednesday. They asked me what our plan was for him and I told them Mom's strong insistence to bring him home. Their recommendation is for him to be in a long-term facility because he needs 24-hour care. They are also concerned for Dad's safety in the care of only Mom and some hired help. Some may say Mom is in denial about what needs to happen. Some may agree that we have to give her a chance to try. Some may think it's too risky to try. I agree with all of them but I think Dad needs to go home - even if it's for a short time. It will give him some closure and a reminder of his real existence. I would want that. If he does have to go to a long-term facility, then at least he had the chance to go home - to say goodbye.

Thursday, March 23rd 2012

Yesterday, I went with Mom to a meeting at the therapeutic treatment residence to discuss plans for Dad's discharge on Wednesday. I'm glad I went. It was necessary for me to be there to help support Mom and her plan for Dad to come home. They came at Mom strongly as they didn't feel she was capable of taking on this task of caring for him. They threw a lot of "What if…" scenarios at her and asked her how she would handle it. I was proud of Mom that day. Her message was clear. It wasn't a matter of how she would do it. It was being brave enough to give Dad the chance. As we've come to realize, other than extra "man power" to care for Dad, this facility doesn't know how to handle him either. His care there is not enough. It may not be enough at home either, but we need to give Dad some closure. The last memory he had at home before his stroke was getting ready in the bathroom so he could go on his morning bike ride. From that point, it's just been a blurry reality for him. He's beginning to show signs of giving up. If he wants to continue living, then he will make it work. If he doesn't, then it's his choice to end this chapter in his life. This is now about giving Dad the choice. Since this whole ordeal started, he hasn't had the choice to make any decisions. The doctors say he is in recovery. He's been in recovery. He will always be in recovery from this day forth. We now need to let him decide the path of his future. There is no doubt this will be the toughest part of this journey.

Sunday, March 25th 2012

I went to visit Dad. He was reading his picture dictionary. I took him out on the patio and handed him a folded paper. I let him struggle with opening it. I've learned that my patience is necessary for his success. It was a March calendar with three days highlighted. I explained slowly to him that this is a reminder and confirmation that he is going home. It was very emotional for him. It appeared he understood. I am anxious and excited for him to come home. No one knows what's to come. Sometimes, it's better that way.

Tuesday, March 27th 2012

I told my students at school that I would not be in tomorrow. I was bringing my dad home. They all looked around at each other and started clapping and smiling. It was heartwarming to know what I do goes beyond just teaching subjects. It's what makes us human. To see empathy in young lives, that's education at its best. No paper, no "A" grade - just real human compassion.

Chapter 2

BRINGING DAD HOME

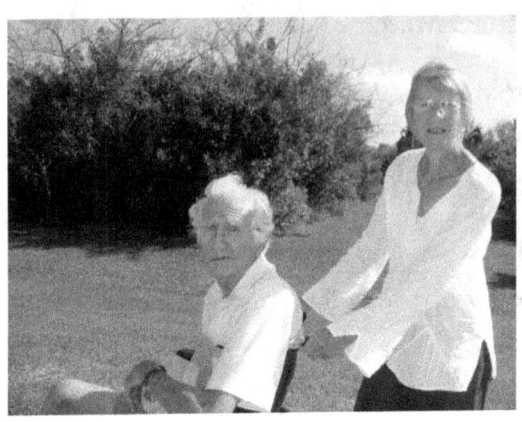

Dad and Mom enjoying the outdoors.

Wednesday, March 28th 2012

Well, it really did happen. Dad came home. I was so glad I was there. It reassured me that we did the right thing. He was thrilled to see his house and all the things in it. He even ate dinner! He also cooperated with us in caring for him. He's going to rest comfortably tonight in a place of peace and quiet. I don't know what tomorrow will bring, but everything we've done so far was worth it. He had his day. He got to come home.

Tuesday, April 3rd 2012

Dad's been home almost a week. We had a wonderful homecoming and birthday party at his house. Mom, Lori and I all have birthdays within a week of each other. We've always celebrated them together. It was great. Dad really is happy to be home. Robin has been staying at Mom's to help her this past week. "Help" does not really explain the job. Mom's been giving everything she has to make this work. It was necessary to have Robin there, not only to help her, but for moral support. But today, Mom wasn't doing well. She was sick to her stomach and not herself at all. It's all catching up with her. I can't imagine what it must be like to be in her shoes right now.

Everyone concerned with Dad's care tells Mom she can't do this. Even the people at the therapeutic treatment center tell her they couldn't do it alone and they are trained. This is not a one man job. We also know that bringing in full-time care will be draining on the bank account. While he was a patient at the center, Dad was giving up. I knew that bringing him home would give him the chance to choose to live or die. Well, he's chosen to live.

Now we are in our next crisis. If we can't work out care for Dad at home and Mom can't manage him without one of us being with her, then this is what we have to consider: Should Mom sacrifice her well-being so that Dad can live, or do we find a nursing home and possibly lose him if he chooses to give up again? This is just too ugly to digest. I am just so thankful that we have a supportive family and we are willing to do whatever it takes. I was dreading Chapter 2. I honestly didn't even know there would be one.

Wednesday, April 4th 2012

Mom's still in a weak state. Therapists, home health care and the social worker have started to make visits to her home. After facing a day of pure exhaustion, Mom has admitted that she can't do this alone. This is a huge step forward for someone as determined and stubborn as she. I hope she doesn't look at this as a failure. If you take a step back, what she did was give Dad the gift to come home. No one else was willing to do that. I have decided to take a week off from work. Robin needs to go home and be with her family. It looks like we need to be careful to not wear ourselves down all at once. I feel so inadequate next to Robin and her caregiving skills. I will do what I have to and maybe my inner strength will come through. God, I hope so.

Thursday, April 5th 2012

I worked my butt off today making school lesson plans so I could take next week off. That was the easy part. Tomorrow, I take over the task of replacing Robin. Dad had a terrible day yesterday. There were long hours of ranting, waving fingers, pushing and resisting any care. We are on the edge of having him "Baker Acted." I hate to use that term but there is nothing safe or good about this situation. If we have to do this, it will allow us to buy some time. We would need to find Dad a full-time facility and Mom needs to get an elder-care attorney to help protect any assets. We're facing the question of: "What is the true quality of life for Dad?" Even if we can control the behavior (which we can't right now), Mom cannot physically continue to care for him at home. I feel we are going against the cycle of life by continuing to tube feed him. Is this really what he wants? Is this really what anyone would want? Who are we kidding? I have a different outlook on death now. I see death as a peaceful place - a place to be with those who have passed before us. A place to have your body and soul back the way it was when life was worth living. Is it awful for me to wish him death? Not on this day.

Sunday, April 8th 2012

Today is Easter. I saw real rabbits hopping through Mom's beautiful lawn at sundown. I've been here three days now. It's difficult to watch Mom try and keep up with Dad's complicated care. There are calm, peaceful times when I think, "This is good. Look how happy Dad is." Other times, I think, "This can't go on. This isn't safe. It's not right." As long as Robin, Lori, or I stay with her, we can allow Dad more time at home. But then what? That time will run out. I thought about the whole aspect of "time" on my jog today. I feel many of us have the need to view time the standard way - looking for a beginning and end to these events we're experiencing.

The clock we are living by has no numbers, no hour hand, or minute hand. It's very unsettling. The truth is no one really knows how much time they have on earth, until they are gone. So all I can do is give the most of my time, where it matters.

Monday, April 9th 2012

The dreaded moment arrived. We knew it would. Mom was just sorry that it came so soon. Dad had another episode last night. He refused his evening meds and tube feeding. He wouldn't remove himself from the kitchen nor even let Mom put him to bed. There was no doubt it was another psychotic event in the making. This wasn't Dad lashing out, afraid, sad, angered, finding blame, and delusional. But it was. Mom was brave enough to make the 911 call. After waiting forty minutes and a standoff in the kitchen with Dad, they arrived, ten of them. There were two or three police and the rest fire rescue/paramedics. There are no words to explain the heartbreak as I listened to Mom pleading in an eerie cry to Dad as they came up the walkway. It was her last attempt to convince him to let her feed him. Even sadder was his lack of acknowledgement of what this meant for him - that his stay at home was coming to a quick end. To our amazement, they didn't know how to handle the situation when they viewed Dad's erratic behavior. They thought his vigorous pointing and words were attached to some true logical thoughts. I sat there stunned and decided to let them figure it out on their own. Eventually, the decision was made to assist Mom with the feeding and meds. The paramedics were not eager to take him to the hospital. They said that once the hospital gives his feeding and meds, Mom and I will have to come pick him up. So they forcefully fed Dad and off to bed he went. All that drama and we didn't accomplish a thing, we didn't buy any extra time.

Tuesday, April 10th 2012

Mom was on board with figuring out a plan for long-term care for Dad. She is so exhausted that it's hard to know how well she is coping and accepting this next step. She made some brave phone calls today to get that going. Tonight we realized that Dad is generally in two states of mind: psychotic or overly medicated. We've tried to find an in-between. There isn't one anymore. It's another sad reality for all involved. Tomorrow, Mom and I will go looking at long-term care facilities. This is a step forward but there's no doubt this will take some searching.

Thursday, April 12th 2012

I was proud of Mom today. She arranged for an aide to come and watch Dad so we could go out and take care of some things. We found a long-term nursing home facility that we liked. It had a nice atmosphere. It was clean, close, and non-hospital like. Mom and I both agreed we would never send Dad back to the therapeutic treatment residence. It was just too awful there. I'll never forget the day Mom was waiting for Dad to use the restroom down the hall. The aide had taken him there and told Mom to wait in the hallway. After waiting some time, Mom got impatient and went in. She found Dad on the bathroom floor. No one was with him. My stomach curdles to think about that incident and the lack of trust Dad experienced with the staff.

Mom filled out the paperwork necessary for registering Dad at the nursing home and took it over to have his doctor sign it. Things seem to be moving in the right direction. I realized today that even when Dad's behavior is under control, it is still not safe for Mom to care for him alone. One day at the house, Mom and I were both on the phone. Not being closely supervised, Dad tried to transfer from his chair to another chair and wound up on the floor. I rushed in when I heard Mom scream. We were both dumbfounded as to what to do with him. We had no idea how to get him up. Eventually, I convinced Mom to let me lift him from behind and we got him back in the chair somehow. Maybe that was my inner strength that I wondered about earlier. It's sad to see how all this is coming together. Dad is making some progress at home and enjoying his surroundings, while Mom is running herself ragged. All the while, we are moving forward in putting Dad back in a long-term facility. I think it will be for good this time. I feel guilty to take away the comfort of home from him. I worry more about how that will affect his recovery. But Mom needs to recover too. She can't go on doing this full time. As I was going to bed last night, I caught a glimpse of the balloon my family brought over for Dad when he came home. It said, "Welcome Back" and it was still hovering.

Friday, April 13th 2012

Today is "Friday the 13th." Mom got a call from the nursing home. They were uncooperative in helping us admit Dad. The bottom line is they don't want him. They don't want to deal with someone so involved, so violent, and on so many medications. We did all that rushing around and now what? The social worker said if they gave us that hard of a time and are not willing to work with us, then we need to look at other places. I guess that beautiful entrance and all the fancy equipment was just for show. They really are just in it for the business and truly don't care. Mom and I gathered ourselves together and decided we will look at more places tomorrow. There's no time for anger and disbelief of another failed attempt.

Mom had hired an elder-care attorney and he hasn't been working out well for us. We think he's been trying to swindle Mom in the worst kind of way. I'm lucky that my siblings have stepped in and started attending some of these meetings with him. It sickens me to see people like him who prey on someone like my mom who is in such need of some real help and guidance.

The court-appointed attorney who was to represent Dad at the guardianship hearing came to Mom's house today. She seemed okay. She was a nice, young professional looking woman. She sat at the table with Dad. We let her experience for herself the responses Dad had to her questions. I think she thought she was going to be able to simply ask some standard questions and get some typical responses. I don't think she was emotionally ready for this. Mom and I didn't intervene by sharing any losses Dad suffered from the stroke or what he could or couldn't do or understand. When she realized she couldn't make sense of any of Dad's speech, she gave him a pen and paper. Dad wrote a mangled looking sentence with no true letters. It had meaning to him though. What it meant, we will never know. She asked Mom what his profession was. Mom told her he was a speech pathologist, audiologist and majored in psychology. Her jaw dropped. I watched her as she tried to compose herself. Our eyes filled with tears as we looked away. Mom and I knew this was not a standard visit for her. Watching her interact with Dad reflected the devastation we were living. She confirmed to Mom that it was not necessary for Dad to be present for the guardianship hearing. It was now obvious to her that Mom should be appointed his guardian. This visit was upsetting for Dad as well. He seems to know quite a bit about what is going on. He shows it through his emotions. I hope Mom will not attempt to have Dad be present at the hearing. Why would anyone want to be in a courtroom, filled with strangers, telling you that you have no more rights to make any decisions in your life? I just can't imagine what good can come from that.

Saturday, April 14th 2012

I had to laugh at some unique moments today. Mom was working so hard to get all of Dad's paperwork together. It's such a consuming job. Out of desperation, she asked Dad if he remembered where his Social Security card was. She'd look at him and point to something. She'd ask, "Here? Is it in here?" Looking at Dad, he had only a blank stare. Then she'd run across the room to something else and go through the whole charades game again. I think Dad found the whole thing amusing. I don't think he grasped the importance of finding his card but I do think he understood Mom's nutty behavior.

Later that day, I went to help Dad out of the bathroom. The house is not wheelchair accessible so he would get stuck quite often. As I was helping him back out, I couldn't help but notice a minty smell in the air and white stuff all down his legs. He had rubbed toothpaste instead of lotion all over his skin. I could bow my head and cry right now, but instead, I'll find humor in it and be glad we got through the day.

Tonight is my last night at Mom's. Tomorrow, I go home. Robin spent a week, I spent a week, and now Lori will spend a week. I think I know now how Robin felt when she left. Torn is a good word. There is still unfinished business of placing Dad in a full-time facility. I feel guilty about leaving this undone. I wish I could stay, but we all have families and it's important that we all go home to them. I'm thankful my sisters and I have been able to rotate our stays with Mom. Lori is coming tomorrow. Since I live nearer to Mom and Dad, I feel that I've been physically and emotionally close with this whole situation. Lori lives in Miami which is a few hours south. I feel she's been more of a support system for me through this. She's learned to listen rather than try and fix everything. That's been helpful. She will undergo living, not hearing, this "reality show." Her past relationship with Dad has not always been good. Although Dad had many faults of his own, I don't think Lori has let go of her hurt feelings. I know how hard it is to forgive someone who has wronged you. I also know how necessary it is to forgive in order to heal a wounded heart.

Thursday, April 19th 2012

During Lori's stay, she did the impossible. She brought the energy and push that the rest of the family had run out of. She took on her well-known in-charge attitude and got Dad admitted to the nursing home that we originally liked. She broke through all the red tape, got things worded correctly, and zipped across town getting the paperwork done. Although this nursing home gave us a hard time the first go-round, it was the right environment for Dad. Lori was able to give Mom some peace of mind by knowing Dad was in a safe place. We couldn't have done this without her.

Chapter 3

UNSPOKEN MESSAGES

Tuesday, April 24th 2012

The court hearing for Mom to take guardianship over Dad is on Thursday. Robin and I will be there for support. Mom seems to be getting back her steam since Dad was admitted to the nursing home. I feel we are all trying to create some space between ourselves and Dad's situation. It can consume you if you let it. I think we've finally shifted from this urgent and anxiety-ridden wish to *save* Dad, to a realization that Dad's recovery will be minimal. We need to accept that and allow him to be given the care he needs. I know what that means for him. It's a huge loss of family life, independence, and the comforts of home. We don't have any choice. He doesn't have any choice. It's just the reality of his health. I wish it didn't have to be this way. I'm proud of Mom for being able to move forward. I know this is a daily struggle for her. She can now focus on taking better care of herself. Something she's put aside for too long.

Thursday, April 26th 2012

Mom received guardianship over Dad today. That was a no-brainer. I was glad Robin and I were there. Before the hearing, Mom's elder-care attorney was rambling off scenarios of finances and situations to Mom. It was out-of-line for him to even attempt to discuss this before the hearing. I could see Mom was not connecting. Her mind was preoccupied with the guardianship, where it should be. When Mom is preoccupied with something, it's so hard for her to concentrate on more than one issue. That's why I was glad we were there. It looks like guardianship and Medicaid don't mesh well. Guardianship looks at a person's assets closely in an attempt to protect that person by making sure any moneys are used for his care. Medicaid will ensure you use all your personal earnings before you ask for government funding. This attorney wants Mom to move money around. Mom wants no part of this. She's told him that. Mom is honest and lives her life that way. We are looking for a new attorney and closing the door on this one. It seems like we will be covering the cost of this expensive journey. That's just the way it is.

Dad now has been moved to the nursing home. It's about 40 minutes from my home. I was visiting him frequently when he was only staying minutes away. Since his move, I haven't been able to see him yet. When I'm thinking about him, I send him little messages from my heart. Positive energy, I guess you'd call it. I hope he gets them.

Friday, April 27th 2012

We are looking at the next decision in front of us. I'm not sure how much Mom has thought about hospice care. I hope we can discuss it when I visit this weekend. I really want Dad to be at peace. I honestly don't think he'll find that wherever he is in this "physical" world anymore. As much as we love Dad, we have to consider his living will. He didn't want this. We shouldn't have allowed that feeding tube to be put in, but it's something we can't go back and change. I believe if you love someone, you have to be willing to let them go. I believe if we allow him to go, he will still be with us - just in spirit. But he will be free of this cruel lifestyle that is so painful for him now. Yes, there is money to keep him alive, but are we doing him justice? Unfortunately, money can't bring him back to whom he was. Can we bring ourselves to accept hospice as the right thing to do? For Dad's sake, I hope so.

Monday, April 30th 2012

Robin and I went to visit Dad at the new nursing home yesterday. I wasn't sure how I would hold up. When we arrived, Dad was sitting away from all the other patients. He immediately became upset upon seeing us. He would point to all the other people in wheelchairs, as if to say, "Look at this, look at what this has come to." I'm really not sure what he's thinking or saying but I know my dad. He doesn't believe he should be there. We took him outside on the patio and he did most of the talking. His eyes spoke, not his words. He is in such a sad place. I tried to cheer him up with my humor but it only lasted for a moment. We all went inside and put together a puzzle of freshwater plants. He was so tired but he pushed on. I'm sure it was one of the few activities that took him away from all the pain. It made him feel normal.

During my visit, I got to know the lady who is stuck in time and thinks her husband is getting new tires for the car. She'd ask the staff, "Where's my husband? He should be here by now!" It became a circling story of being locked in a senseless moment in her life. I also watched as another lady would coddle a baby doll. She held it as though it was real. It showed the small comforts of an artificial life. It's heartbreaking everywhere you look. I'm not sure how my visit affected Dad. I think family can be comforting yet disturbing in this situation. I'm still glad I went to visit him. He's in the loneliest place in his life right now.

I talked with my neighbor Marie today. She's lost quite a few loved ones and had some interesting insight. I mentioned to her that on my visit I noticed there were only a few men compared to women at the facility. She looked at me with knowing eyes and said that men don't last long in that situation. Many stop eating and wither away. They don't want to be there and quickly end things on their own. She told me they don't feel hunger like we do. Hunger is not painful when you're in that transition. I think that's why Dad is so tired and sad. The feeding tube is not allowing him to make that choice.

Sunday, May 6th 2012

I drove up to Mom's house and had a good conversation with her. We talked about Dad openly and we shared our thoughts about his condition, his behavior, his whole situation. Mom made a generalization that everyone else who lives at the facility is like a potted plant. I found that humorous but quite true - everyone but Dad. They are all so passive and calm. It's like they have accepted this last chapter of their life. Not Dad. He still has bouts of anger and lashes out at Mom on some visits. Mom told me she reassured Dad that he needs to be brave; that she was taking care of all the bills and that a judge was watching over him. To some that may sound reassuring but to a person like Dad, or any man who took primary care of his family, it could be downright humiliating. I know Mom didn't mean it to be like that. I've just gained a lot of experience of viewing things from different perspectives.

After visiting Mom, I went to see Dad. It was difficult for me to walk through those doors and just as difficult to leave. I have to remember that Dad can't do that. He has to stay. And that's more difficult than anything I have to do. I brought Skippy with me. It was the first time Dad has seen him since he left home. He held him and gave him kisses. It was a nice moment.

"I CEZ LIFE." That's what I was left with upon leaving Dad today. His writing wasn't clear and neither was the message. Just like his language, I wonder if the words match his thoughts at all. He wrote so intently, making sure I saw it before I left. As I tried reading it back to him, I didn't get any feeling from him that I understood or interpreted it correctly. So I left him with a verbal, "I love you." I always repeat it twice and he finishes the last word.

I wonder what it was that Dad was trying to write before I left? I think one day I'll know - just not today.

Chapter 4

THE NEXT SIX MONTHS

Saturday, May 12th 2012

Yesterday, Mom took Dad to see his neurologist. I'm proud of her for following through with his appointment. It's a challenge getting him to the doctor. She got a medical van to help take him there. There are so many things to worry about. But as I look back at Dad's recent behavior, it was critical to get his medications adjusted. His visit provided some much needed information. As Mom got Dad through the entrance door, he had one of his episodes. According to Mom, he was wailing, protesting, and lashing out. These are the typical behaviors we have been seeing. The doctor was able to witness this and Dad now has a new diagnosis pseudobulbar affect. It's a syndrome from brain injury where one loses the ability to control emotions.

So to sum up his disability, he had a cerebrovascular accident (stroke) which left him paralyzed on his right side. Due to the stroke he also has the condition aphasia, which is caused by brain injury. It is the loss of the ability to communicate verbally or use written words. It affects the ability to speak, read, write, recognize the names or pictures of objects, or understand what other people have said. He also has some degree of agnosia which is loss of memory for the use of common objects. For example, sometimes he picks up an empty glass and tries to pour it into the thickened juice container. He suffers from incontinence, psychotic depression that is progressively worsening, dementia, chronic hematuria (blood in the urine), stage three renal failure, and now with pseudobulbar affect. Plus he's taking eight medications to treat cholesterol, blood pressure, anxiety, pain, depression, stomach ulcers, delusions, and a blood thinner to prevent another stroke. This is getting harder by the day to think that Dad's quality of life is worth living. I'm having a hard time looking at the big picture. With all that he has lost, he now has one more diagnosis on top of it all. This is just unreal.

Mom is so involved with being a guardian that I'm afraid she's overlooking Dad's quality of life. I think an intervention is in the near future. I look back to when my dog, Cane, was near the end of his road. He wasn't able to see well, go for walks anymore, and control his bladder. He was in pain and I knew it. I now think it was selfish of me to let it go on for so long. I don't want that for Dad. Mom wants to do what's right. She'll sacrifice everything for his well-being. I hope she soon sees Dad's degree of suffering. It's our responsibility to make decisions in his best interest. This realization will take some time. Mom has to be on board with this, so she needs time to get there. It's hard to be patient, but it's necessary.

I often think about Dad during the day. I feel that I am grieving the death of someone who hasn't died yet. When I'm alone, I seem to relate to him in spirit. Like someone who has already passed on. I think I do this because I want to remember him in a better light than now. I want him to be at peace. I hope for that. I feel his true being is no longer here.

When I went to see him today, I found fewer connections within our conversation. I don't know if it's because of the strong medications he's on or the true deterioration of his condition. It may be both. It gets harder every visit. I wish I could say something to comfort him, but I'm out of words. I have nothing to inspire him to pull through. He can't come home. That used to be the driving force. So what do you say to someone … my father … now? I can only stare into his eyes and hold his hand.

Friday, June 1st 2012

It's been a while since I've spilled my heart on these pages. I've found some peace knowing Dad is being well cared for at the nursing home. That doesn't mean his condition is any better. It just means that I'm able to sleep at night again. I feel at ease knowing Mom feels the same way.

On Memorial Day weekend, Robin, Lori and I visited Dad together. We also had a much needed conversation with Mom about hospice. I could see the wall she was putting up. She even mentioned bringing Dad home again. None of us could understand that bizarre comment. We told her neither his doctor nor we would support that. We've already tried having Dad home. Mom's health and safety was of great concern during that time. I was worried for Mom and felt she was headed for a nervous breakdown. We talked about hospice and she had the typical assumption that hospice was for when a person is dying. We tried to explain to her that hospice is there to support her as she goes through this difficult process. They are there to help manage pain for the patient rather than the defeated attempt of physical therapy. I hope she heard some of what we said. Listening to her, however, allowed me to understand - to see where she is on this journey.

The other night Lori had a conversation with Mom and told her that Dad's rejection and violent behavior toward her is his way of disconnecting himself. It's what people and animals do when they are ready to die. It's a natural process that she shouldn't take personally. She told Mom that she needs to distance herself from him as well. She should not give up on him but respect this natural process. As harsh sounding as that is, I think she's right. I'm glad she's a part of this family. I don't know that I could be that strong and tell things so matter-of-factly.

On my next visit with Dad, I want to tell him that if he's okay with living out his life in this condition, then I will support him. I also want to tell him that if he's ready to pass on, that his children are all okay with that too. The hardest part will be not knowing if he understands my words. I may not be able to have the courage to say these things to him, but my thoughts confirm where I am on this journey as well.

Wednesday, June 5th 2012

Tomorrow is Dad's birthday. He will be 82 years old. I plan to drive and see him. This is another difficult day to understand in my dad's world. I've talked with my family and we all agreed to keep his birthday low-keyed. We decided not to mention it unless he seems to know. The reasoning is sad. Who wants to recognize their birthday when they are in a condition like his? I think it would be almost cruel to bring attention to it. Yet, this may be his last one. No one knows for sure. I'll try my best to make it special. I'll share the news of my new position as the art teacher next year. I'll hold his hand and wish him a silent "Happy Birthday." I'll be there for him. I know that is the best gift I could give.

Thursday, June 7th 2012

Today was Dad's birthday. I went to visit him as planned. I thought about what to bring. I ended up bringing some cut-up watermelon. That's all, nothing to acknowledge his birthday. When I arrived at 10 a.m., he was napping. When he woke up, he seemed happy to see me. After a few minutes, the crying set in. To try and break him from this crying spell, I shared news of what was going on in my life. He would pause and stop crying for a moment. Just as quickly, it would start up all over again. I tried to be strong, but it didn't last long. I gave him a big hug and we had a good cry together. At least he wasn't alone.

Thirty minutes had passed and I felt I was doing more harm than good by being present. So I attempted to get him up out of bed and out of his room. Since it had started raining, I suggested going out to the main room to do the ocean puzzle that we had done a few times before. As we started on the puzzle, I reassured myself that not mentioning his birthday was the right thing to do. He was in no state of mind to take this on. We ate a little watermelon and placed a few puzzle pieces together.

A few minutes later, I noticed some family members gathering around one of the patients. I then hear, "Let's all sing together! Happy Birthday to you ..." and so it went. A huge sensation of guilt came over me. I slowly and cautiously lifted my head to look up at Dad's expression. There was none. He didn't make any connection to the song, or that people were gathering for someone else's birthday celebration or that it was his own birthday. I felt terrible. To make matters worse, a nice lady offered us cake. I declined. Just when I thought I had survived this awful moment, another visitor entered the main room. She told the group next to me she was sorry she had missed the singing. So they sang the whole song again for her. I couldn't believe I had to relive this twice. Dad became upset and started crying again but I don't believe it was connected to the singing. The aides looked over and saw Dad upset and gave me a look of, "I'm sorry." They had no idea how hard this was for me. I came up to see my dad on his birthday and I couldn't wish my own father a happy birthday. I took my dad's hand, held it tight, and wished him a happy birthday in thought.

The rain had finally stopped, so we went out on the patio. We could smell the rain on the sidewalk; we could feel the thick air from the humidity, and we could see the greyness of the day as the clouds kept the sun from glaring. It was beautiful. We strolled by the trees and stopped at the gazebo. It was quiet, peaceful, and Dad was now calm. He would utter sounds as he looked at the landscaping. I started to doze off as we enjoyed the silence together. As I opened my eyes, knowing I was falling asleep, Dad was looking at me. He was enjoying watching me. I don't know what he was thinking but I know he was in a good place for the moment. Then we wheeled through some puddles and made our way back inside. I gave Dad lots of hugs and kisses. I told him I loved him and that I would see him soon. He was teary again. Upon leaving, I have to go through two security coded locked doors. I broke down before I got out the second door. "Happy Birthday, Dad."

Thursday, June 14th 2012

The psychiatrist at the nursing home is concerned about Dad. He has lost 7 lbs. in a week. He has stopped eating by mouth and is only taking two out of the usual four of his tube-feedings. It was mentioned to Mom if she had considered taking out the feeding tube. I was glad someone else had finally spoken up. By Mom's reaction, as guardian, she didn't seem to think this was a decision she had permission to make. I know Dad is suffering. He is going to have to fight to get to the other side. I wish it didn't have to be so hard, especially for Mom. I think the emotional strings she has tied to him are wound too deeply. I also think she feels an obligation as his guardian to keep him alive. This is a different role for her than making life decisions as his wife. It shouldn't be, but it is. She can't see this from the point of view of the rest of the family. This is a hard place for her to be right now.

Next week, all my siblings will be here. Darrow is coming from Tokyo, Robin is coming to help with Dad's doctor's appointment and Lori said she'd come for support. I think this is our opportunity as a family to tell Mom to let go; that we are all here for her and that it's the right thing to do. We need to stop anymore life-saving measures. We want Dad to be at peace. I hope Mom will see that and let us love and support her to the end.

Sunday, June 17th 2012

Dear Dad,

Today is Father's Day. Sunday, June 17th, 2012. Many people find cards a way to sum up how they feel. I feel that many cards leave out a whole lot. Let my poem explain.

Father's Day

A card can't hold your hand the way I can.

A card can't gaze into your eyes and give you a warm smile the way I can.

A card can't remind you of how I'd sit on your lap as a child and say, "Candy, Daddy? Candy?"

A card can't thank you for capturing so much of our lives through pictures.

A card can't remind you of your passion for jogging and how you instilled exercise in our lives at such a young age.

A card can't thank you for supporting me and providing the finances to go to college and become an educated adult.

A card can't remind you of how supportive you were for the choices I made in my life, like marrying my husband Dave.

A card can't tell you the laughter you would bring with all your jokes.

A card can't thank you for being a part of my children's lives and supporting them at Honor Roll and promoting all their talents in music and sports.

A card can't tell you that you were, are, and will always be a loving father.

A card can't tell you that I love you enough to let you go when you are ready. That I want you to find peace and comfort again. That I know you will always be with me, looking down on me, and still being there to enjoy the wonders of my life and to comfort me in difficult times. A card can't tell you how much I love you Dad.

Happy Father's Day.

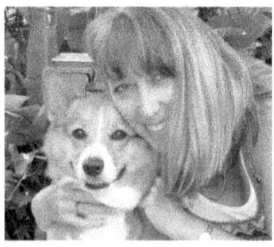

Love your daughter, Aimi

I tried to rehearse my poem one line at a time aloud on my drive up to see Dad today. I couldn't do it. My emotions would take over and I'd have to start over again. After many attempts, I didn't think I'd get to read this to Dad. I put it away in my bag and decided to see if I was brave enough to pull it out during my visit. When I got to Mom's house, she decided to come along and bring Skippy. I was happy about that since most of my visits to Dad were solo.

When we arrived, to our surprise, Dad was eating his lunch. He ate the meat and potatoes; even ate some carrots and half of his cheese cake. So for someone who has lost 7 lbs., this is another peculiar moment that just confuses us all. We joined Dad for lunch and then went out to the patio. I brought some new puzzles. Mom brought the CD player and Skippy who was the perfect lap dog for Dad. Mom gave Dad a haircut and filed his nails. After some time, Mom hinted that she was ready to go. I hadn't read my poem yet. I hadn't planned on Mom being present either. I told her to wait and pulled it out. I handed it to Dad and told him it was something I had written for him for Father's Day. He was unaware that it was Father's Day. I let him take it out of the envelope and he looked at it intently, as if he was reading it. I'll never know for sure if he was. Mom was right behind him reading it to herself. She was mouthing the words as tears rolled down her face. She became extremely emotional. I asked Dad if I could read my poem to him and so I did. With many pauses and deep breaths, I got through it. I had told Dad why I loved him. I had said goodbye before it was too late. He now knew that I would be strong when he needed to be weak. I had accepted his death beforehand and I had the courage to tell him that it would be okay. I'm glad I read the poem. It was one of the hardest things I've ever done.

Tuesday, June 26th 2012

What a week. Darrow came in town with his family, Lori came up and Robin and my niece, Justine, came down. It was good to have everyone together. Dad had lots of visits with family. He seemed to enjoy all the attention.

We teamed up to help get Dad to his neurologist appointment. That was no easy task. To get someone in Dad's condition ready on time and hope he is cooperative is asking a lot. I'm glad Mom didn't have to do it alone.

We are still trying to get Mom to involve hospice. I think she is starting to understand where we are coming from and the need to plan for the next stage of Dad's journey. Robin, Lori and Darrow helped to end all ties with the attorney who was supposed to help Mom with the guardianship and budget. It leaves a bad taste in your mouth when you realize someone was trying to take advantage of Mom when she was in such a fragile state and needed to trust in order to get this done. These few days really showed how strong we are as a family unit, each with different strengths, but all critical in the support system for Mom. We found a new elder-care attorney and now feel that the budget will be submitted to the judge. We can now move forward.

When I called Mom today, she was visiting with Dad on the patio. She handed the phone to Dad. I told him what I was cooking for dinner and all the small tasks I was doing. He parroted much of the conversation back to me. For a moment it was quite eerie. I felt I was talking to a young child - trying to keep the wording slow and simple. It just seems so full circle. It doesn't feel right.

Friday, June 29th 2012

I will be leaving town with my family for a vacation to the Keys for two weeks. I'm nervous about leaving for that length of time. I decided to also take my car on the trip in case something were to happen while I'm gone. Anxiety weighs heavily on me about leaving but I know I can't put my life on hold or my family's for much longer.

I went to visit Dad today. I also brought Skippy whom he loves. When I got there, it was evident he wasn't having a good day. My visit seemed to really help calm him down and comfort him. That's also the benefit of bringing the dog. There's nothing more healing than unconditional love from an old friend.

During our visit on the patio, I would say certain things to see if Dad remembered our last visit together. I told him I was going to be the art teacher next year. I looked at his expression. He looked surprised as though this was news to him. So I told him all over again. Although he couldn't remember this from before, I didn't mind telling him again and seeing his excitement for me. During one of his intense conversations with me (subject unknown), he used a word I hadn't heard him use and one I haven't used in front of him either - "Heaven."

Friday, July 6th 2012

I'm in the Keys vacationing with my family. Mom has my dog, Flounder, whom I miss. Yet, I am enjoying the freedom of not having to worry about him for a change. This trip has allowed me to reflect on things in my life. I'm reading a book called, "Final Gifts" by Maggie Callanan and Patricia Kelly. It's a book about understanding the special awareness, needs, and communications of the dying. I haven't put it down yet. It is incredibly interesting. It focuses on many aspects that all the family members involved experience. The only thing that makes our situation with Dad a little different is his lack of language. Although because of the stroke, I wonder how much of it would make sense if he *had* the language.

I've realized how Dad's stroke has truly affected my wellbeing. You go through something like this and try to make yourself strong and less important in the scheme of things. Well, I sure paid the price. After a dental checkup and two consecutive visits for cavities, I found there was a price to pay for my negligence. I also discovered that I was grinding my teeth terribly. I had a night guard made and now realize that three months of neck pain and occasional morning headaches were all due to the stress of me grinding my teeth - more guilt.

I also have done lots of internet research on art to help me prepare for my new teaching position this fall. I brought a bag of art supplies on this trip. I brought them down to the beach while the boys were out fishing. It's very hard to get back into this after feeling my creative side had been shut down for so long. As I got enough courage to draw, I noticed a boat coming. I quickly put my art pad back in my bag because I thought it was my family approaching. This jerk reaction made me realize my insecurity of my own ability. It also made me realize that I have a lot of work ahead of me. I need to push through this and gain some confidence. My art work exposes who I am. I feel like a hermit crab without it's shell. I think this year is going to teach me more about myself. I hope it will help reveal the side of me that's been hidden for so long.

Tuesday, July 17th 2012

Now back from vacation, I took the boys to Mom's house. The plan was to cut her grass while I visited Dad. That plan changed as the skies turned grey and the summer storms rolled in. Mom suggested that I take the boys to visit Dad since they hadn't seen him in almost six months. I was reluctant because a part of me doesn't feel it's necessary for them to feel the emotional pain, as I do, visiting him each week. I want them to remember Dad as the joking grandpa and the music buff that he was. But with a little guilt from Mom saying that it could be the last time, I let the boys decide. So Drew, Jonny, and Skippy came with me in the pouring rain. It turned out to be a nice visit. I think the anxiety of not knowing how the visit will go is the worst part. Dad was happy to see them and blew them his loving kisses. We spent lunch time talking about our trip to the Keys. I asked Dad if he remembered that I was going to be the art teacher next year, and he did.

I didn't cry when I left. Surprisingly, I was emotionally okay. The boys were brave. I think this visit allowed them to see other people who are at the end of their journey as well. It's sad, but maybe they will cherish the time they have left with their other grandparents while they still have their good health.

Saturday, September 1st 2012

It's been a while since I've written my thoughts about Dad. I still visit him but it's about every two weeks now. I've started back at work so things have been busy on the weekends. For some time, I thought that Dad would make improvements, decline or go up and down as he had in the past. It turns out that this last month he's mostly been stable. Mom seems to be able to continue to visit him daily with him being accepting of her visits. No perfect report card but much better than past visits.

Today, Skippy and I went to see Dad. I joined him for lunch and then a visit on the patio. He still recognizes me but his eyes are different. They use to be full of emotion and thoughts. It was like I could look into them and see behind his outer shell, even if his words made no sense. But now his eyes are not as clear. They are visibly less bright and somewhat hazy. I only catch small glimpses of a real connection.

Dad started singing while we were outside. A very soft, mumbled rhythm, but he was singing. We sang "Blue Bayou" and "Raindrops Keep Falling on my Head." When he sings, he can actually mouth the right words. I could see this was pleasurable for him. It also made him sad - me too. There are moments I see him so trapped when I look in his eyes. There is nothing I can say other than, "I'm here for you." When I was leaving, he pulled on my bag. I knew what that meant. I didn't make it out the front entrance without crying.

I've realized that I am just the support system. Mom will continue to let this go on if she truly believes she should. Mom's heart always gets the best of her no matter how realistic we (the children) are about Dad's quality of life and taking the next step. There isn't much more I can do but be there for them. (I hate watching sad movies.)

Thursday, September 27th 2012

Robin came down and Lori came up this past weekend. We all went to visit Dad. He's been terribly resistant to

Mom lately. She often thinks he blames her for his situation and for keeping him there. He was okay with us. It makes your stomach turn when you walk in and look to see where he is. We found him at the end of the hallway, backed into the corner with his head slouched over. Once he saw us, he made lots of "oh" sounds. He really enjoyed listening to the three of us chat out on the patio. When it was time to leave, he peeked through the small window in the door as we left. It's so hard to turn around and see him on the other side. It's even harder to look and wave - another teary exit for us all.

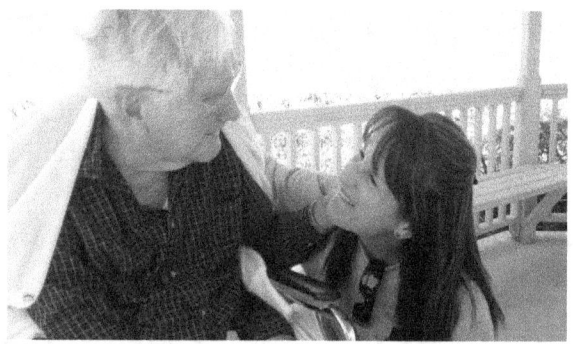

Dad and Robin in the gazebo.

I sometimes hope that one day, on the other side, I'll be able to have a real conversation with Dad again. I really wish I could hear what he's thinking and console him in some way. It's just that hard.

Monday, October 8th 2012

Since Dad's stroke, I really thought this whole deal was about him. Now I know differently. The family involved is also a patient. They just don't get the spotlight, the monitoring of doctors, the strong medications and the cooked meals. Dad is just a piece of this large network of misery.

Yesterday, I went on my Sunday voyage to see Dad. They increased his medication due to his recent more aggressive behavior and crying spells. He seemed to be in the same state of mind as usual. He was a little overly emotional but not to any extreme. He was manageable. In his unrecognizable language, he told me how miserable he was. I don't need to identify any words to know this.

Then we looked at my wedding album. I read to him a speech he wrote and read at my wedding. He listened so intently to his use of Shakespearian styled phrases and his choice to use vocabulary that most people would have to look up. To both of us, it was poetic and musical. It was a wonderful feeling to hear something from him that was truly meant for me. This is something I don't expect to happen anymore. He enjoyed looking at the pictures and still remembers how he hated the mustache that he had during the wedding. We had lunch together and he accompanied me to the door. He gave me a kiss goodbye and watched me walk away. I thought it was a successful visit because I didn't cry when I left.

I went back to Mom's house to take Skippy home and to see if she needed me to help with anything. We sat in the living room and chatted like we always do when I return. I told her about my visit. She then showed me all the paperwork she'd been working on and where she keeps it in case anything was to ever happen to her. This is a common thing now. She's ridding the house of clutter, giving us kids all the special notes from our childhood, asking us to take any of the trinkets and such that have been sitting on her shelves for all these years. She's been acting like she's dying.

During our discussion she talks of other women who are left to take care of their spouses. She tells me about one woman who would come to visit her husband. Mom said she hadn't seen her in a few weeks. Then one day she showed up in a wheelchair with her grown child. She had injured her hip. After a few of these stories, Mom says as she's said before, "If I can only outlive Dad. That's all I need to do." Then she says it again but adds, "If I can only outlive Dad, then I'm out of here." I said, "What do you mean you're out of here?" She says again, "I'm out of here" and points up.

Chapter 5

HOPELESSNESS, HOPE, AND HEROES

Friday, October 13th 2012

Mom called me at work around 2 p.m. This was disturbing because she doesn't usually call me at this time. Something wasn't right. She said Dad had been running a fever since last night. The doctor had run tests and couldn't figure out why. They also did a chest x-ray, blood work, urine check, and were now waiting for a culture to come back. That was enough for me to decide to leave work early so I could be there.

When I finally got on the expressway, I was stuck in traffic from a prior accident. That added about an hour to my commute. I felt trapped as I sat there. I kept thinking, "There must be a reason why this is happening." Knowing I had no control over the situation, I had to accept that this plan was greater than me. I just need to stop questioning it.

After an hour and a half, I finally arrived. Dad was in his wheelchair out on the patio with Mom. He was his "normal" self. Dad had miraculously come back to life. Mom looked at me dumbfounded. I sat with him and he gave me his traditional speech about how awful things were (in his language). I just held his hand and listened.

As I was talking with him, he couldn't remember that I visited him last weekend. I showed him pictures of my wedding again. Even though he couldn't remember looking at the album before, I know it was meaningful and mattered at the time. I could see how happy he was to see me and be with me.

When a doctor says there is an infection, the patient is running a fever, and nobody knows why… this is where I start to believe that this is part of the greater plan. I think this was a sign of things to come. I don't know how many more there will be but it doesn't matter, as long as I'm there.

After my visit with Dad, I went back to Mom's house and got to spend some time with her. We went for a nice long bike ride around the neighborhood. While riding, I was thinking about Mom. She asks for so little but needs so much.

That evening, I went home and sat in my therapeutic hot tub. I haven't spent much time in there lately. It's a great place for me to think and figure things out. After a few minutes, I found myself pleading with God as if there was a check list. Everything is checked off. We are all, so I think, ready to let Dad pass. I have said my good-byes. I have vowed to take care of Mom. I have prayed to let this happen in the most caring and humane way possible. As much as I begged for a sign to let Dad go, I felt that God had already given it. I felt in my heart that the fever was a way to draw Mom and me near to say goodbye. Maybe he wants to die alone. I just don't know.

I've been writing another poem. I do that when emotions run deep.

Be Free

Trying so hard,
With all my might,
To understand,
This course of life.

I find myself pleading
With God,
To raise you,
Ever so gently,
Weightless,
Leaving behind,
This broken shell.

Taking,
Only He,
Can mend the pieces of you,
Of what time,
Here on earth,
Cannot.

You taught me,
Spoken language,
Needs only rhythms and patterns.
Eyes,
Speak louder than words.
Emotions,
Run deep.
Trying to share your message,
Let the truth be told.

Your illness,
A calling,
A message,
A warning,
I'm at ease.

We'll take care of Mom,
We'll hold her hand,
Guiding her,
Until she lets go.
Be free.

Don't mind my selfishness,
Of missing you,
You will be with me,
Everlasting.

You'll be,
That warm breeze,
Under a tree.
That song bird,
Off in the distance.
That squirrel,
That stops for a moment,
Rather than prancing away.
That warm feeling of comfort,
When I need my dad.

I'll find you,
In the beauty of life.
Let go,
Embrace the light.
Be free.

Wednesday, October 24th 2012

Last weekend, I went to see Dad. Mom joined me on the visit. I'm not really sure why. I like to go with the intention of giving Mom a day off. She goes every day even though we recommend that she not go so often. It takes such a toll on her. Now it's part of her routine. Good or bad, she's there. I think she went with me because it recreates a scenario of "family"- something that she only has in bits and pieces these days. Don't get me wrong. We are there for Mom more now than ever. But living by yourself in a big empty house paints a lonely picture. I'm glad she went with me. It turned out to be a nice visit.

Just this week Dave's parents, Bill and Evelyn, went to visit Dad for the first time. Mom had asked them to come up. Mom said the visit went fine. Dad was very teary eyed. He recognized them as he does most everyone. They sat on the patio and looked at pictures. Bill and Evelyn bragged about the grandchildren they all share. Mom said she walked them out and then came back to get Dad's dirty laundry. She said Dad was having a fit about something. He was yelling and carrying on. He even got so frustrated that he began hitting his head with his hand. This was the first time I've heard of this behavior. It was another episode according to Mom. I continually ask myself and God: "How much is too much?"

When I talked to Bill and Evelyn after their visit, they said their visit to see Dad was extremely difficult for them. They had never seen Dad in this state. Mom and I are accustomed to seeing Dad this way. It's difficult for anyone to visit him, especially because of his lack of speech. The visitor has to do most of the talking and then be strong enough to listen to Dad's incomprehensible response. I feel bad asking anyone to go through this.

Thursday, October 25th 2012

During my daily call to Mom, I always ask how Dad is. She said she had a really nice visit. She brought an old photo album as she usually does. All Dads' life, he spent it capturing our family in pictures. He worked so hard to get all the photos in albums. We have shelves lined with them, all in order. I never thought that he would benefit the most from them. He remembers things from long ago if he has a picture. This is the only way to retell his life to him. This particular album went way back in time. Dad tried to open it backwards. Mom did her best to redirect him to start from the front. As he opened the cover, taped to the inside was something Mom never expected to find - his Social Security card. All she could do was laugh. Dad laughed along with her, as though he knew it was there all along. He was the one who hid it there. It took her back to that day when we had brought him home and she was pleading with him to tell her where it was. Some things, I just don't understand. I'm glad they got a good laugh out of it.

Saturday, November 3rd 2012

While I was out running errands around noon, I received a call from Mom. I knew she visits Dad at that time. That meant I was going to talk with Dad on the phone. After a brief "Hello" from Mom, I hear: "Here's Dad." I proceed to have a conversation with him. I do all the talking and I pretend his mumbled replies are a response I understand. His voice is only faintly familiar as Dad's old voice. It no longer has the excitement or the tone it did when we would talk before his stroke. I can only pretend to have one of our old conversations. It's sad and hard to do, but I do it. I'm thankful no one else was in the car. These moments are very uncomfortable for me. I don't like sharing these calls in the presence of others because when I do, it validates to everyone listening just how much my dad has lost.

Mom called me later that afternoon to tell me how sick it made her feel to see the bank statements and bills for Dad's care. It costs eighteen thousand dollars for two months of care and medications. It's been ten months since Dad's stroke. I think Mom is finally beginning to see a piece of the big picture. There is a huge price to pay to keep Dad alive. My thoughts on this are not blinded by a lifelong emotional bond. To me, it makes no difference if we spend $10 or $8,000 a month on Dad. It isn't whether he is in a nursing home or living at home. It's his quality of life. We have made the choices to keep Dad alive these last ten months. Aren't we ultimately responsible for this? If it were not for the heavy medications and the feeding tube, he would not be with us. So how do we get Mom to see this? At what point will Mom realize that her love and all her efforts won't change this situation? How much longer can we bear the pain of watching Dad go through this? Mom's been running the show. Our attempts to help her make any changes have failed. We don't want to wait until she hurts herself or falls ill and can no longer make these decisions. I wish, and hope to God, she can find the courage to move forward.

Monday, November 19th 2012

It's a few days before Thanksgiving. I went with Mom to visit Dad today. We had a non-eventful visit for lunch. What a relief.

On my drive home, I started thinking about where I was last year. A year ago, Mom called me to tell me we couldn't have Thanksgiving at her house. She said Dad wouldn't be able to handle it. Having Thanksgiving at my house was not a problem. The reason we couldn't have it at Mom and Dad's house was the problem. After a few phone calls to Mom and some probing, my sisters and I came to realize that Dad had hurt Mom. She said he got into a rage and pushed her against the stove. She struck back in defense and scratched him. At that point, I jumped in my car to see for myself what had happened. When I arrived, Dad was riding the lawn mower. I was on the brink of a battle. Dad saw me strut right past him to find Mom who was also working in the yard. I told Mom to show me what happened. She had some bruising on her arms and a few scratches. She told me her side of what happened. She said she brought this on herself. When she said that, I knew she was the victim here. Dad soon approached and asked what was going on. I verbally lashed out at him. I don't usually lose my cool and talk to him like this, but I did that day. He denied ever laying a hand on her. He denied everything. He even blamed Mom for the scratches on his arms. I told Mom she shouldn't stay. She could stay with any of us. She told me that she loved him and that they would get through this. She wasn't leaving. I swore to Dad that if he ever laid another hand on her, I'd call the police.

It was the worst feeling in the world to see my Dad crying, defending himself and me possibly having to cut him off from my family. I left that day with the most sickening feeling I've ever felt. I also knew that if Dad didn't get help and, if Mom wouldn't leave, this was going to get worse. I feared for Mom's life.

We had Thanksgiving at my house that year. Mom came but Dad stayed home. Between that event and ending the year 2011, I somehow found some forgiveness for Dad. I needed to. I knew life was too short. I wanted him to see his grandchildren. I wanted my dad in our life.

On January 3rd, approximately one month later, he had his stroke. I believe this stroke saved Mom's life. I look back now and see the signs of dementia. Dad was someone who needed help long before this. Now we are coming full circle. Again, Thanksgiving will be at my house with all the family but Dad will remain at the nursing home. I can't believe what has truly gone on this past year. I believe writing all this down, the raw and ugly truth, will be an important part of surviving.

Tuesday, November 27th 2012

Thanksgiving has come and gone. We had a pleasant meal with Mom and the family. It was nice to see my sisters and get some of the cousins together.

We spent the next day at Mom's house clearing out overgrown bushes. The property is overwhelming for her. She has two acres and a pool to maintain by herself now. I'm not sure how long she'll be able to keep up with it. I imagine if she can maintain her health, she will stay there and sell it when Dad passes.

The following day we went to visit Dad with all our children. I knew this would be hard. It was disturbing for everyone, especially the kids. The look on Jonny's face said it all. He could see the pain and sadness Dad was expressing. I was proud of the boys. They all came together and did this for Dad. I know it meant so much to him but I also think it broke his heart. It made him realize how much he misses out on.

Once everyone left, I broke down. It was time. You can only be strong for so long. After a good cry and a long walk, I again dug for that inner strength. I'll keep digging for as long as it takes.

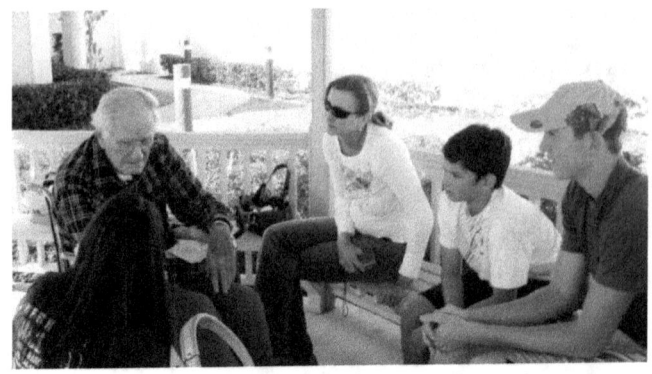

From left: Robin, Dad, Lori, Jonny, and Austin

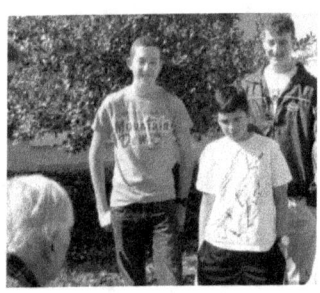

From left: Dad, Kyle, Jonny, and Noah

Monday, December 17th 2012

Last Friday was a tremendous step for Mom. She had finally set up a meeting with a hospice counselor. Robin, Lori, Darrow and I were able to be there to support her. All of us have been waiting for this meeting to happen for a long time. We just had to wait patiently until Mom was ready. I had suggested to Robin, a few weeks prior, to write a letter that briefly states Dad's condition and his eligibility for hospice. She's familiar with all the medical terms and also Dad's condition, which is so complex. I told her all the children would sign it. Then Mom could have it. She would have a written document that basically says: "We are all with you. You are not alone." When the time comes, or when she is ready, she will know that this was a decision we all made together. Robin said she mentioned the idea to Mom during Thanksgiving, so I wonder if that helped Mom to take this step to meet with hospice.

The meeting was very informative. The hospice counselor helped to clarify Mom's rights as Dad's guardian. Now they will move forward and assess Dad for eligibility. Before Darrow goes back to Tokyo, we plan to come together again and meet with the counselor from the nursing home who can help to be an advocate for Mom. We hope to reduce some of the tube feedings so Dad can make the choice to eat. There is so much resistance from the nursing home to change anything with Dad. They consider him stable. If he can take in food, whether it's from a tube or by mouth, and his body doesn't reject it, he is stable. He is physically stable. They don't look at the emotional or mental stability. He has to be highly medicated all the time just to be manageable. We see the pain and sadness Dad faces each day. We see his loss to interpret much of the language spoken around him. We see the immediate loss of memory from the prior day. We see his inability in all facets of his life.

Noah, my teenage nephew, had an interesting viewpoint during one of our visits. He said, "Isn't *living* the ability to create new memories?" After thinking about it, I was left speechless. I guess it just depends whom you ask.

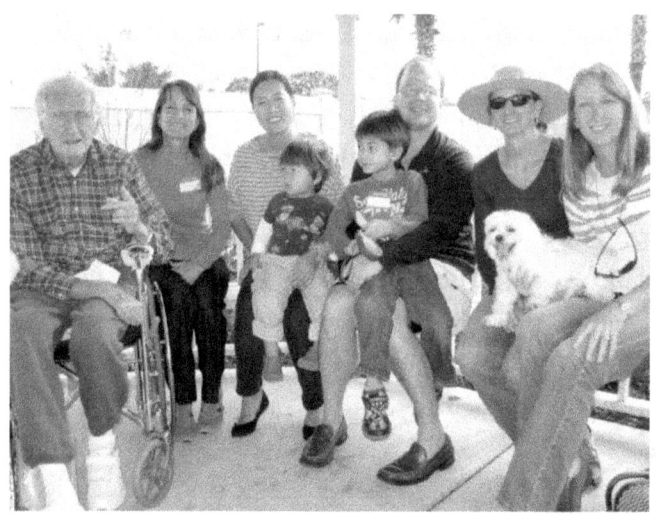

From left: Dad, Robin, Hisako, Alex, Darrow Jr., Darrow, Lori, Skippy and Aimi

Thursday, December 20th 2012

Hospice came for the eligibility meeting for Dad. Mom met them at the nursing home to observe. After their analysis, they said Dad doesn't qualify at this time. He meets everything on all the checklists except one box. The box that states that the doctor says he has a six-month life expectancy. The hospice representative felt Dad was still suffering from deep depression and said she would recommend that his medication be increased. Mom met with Dad's doctor the next day while passing him in the hallway. He asked how the meeting went and about Dad's results of being accepted into hospice. According to Mom, he was genuinely concerned by the results but understood that Dad did not meet the six-month life expectancy. He told Mom that Dad is on the brink. He didn't explain further about what he meant by that comment. He also didn't want to reduce his tube feedings. This is not the first time Mom has requested this. He said there are moral and ethical obligations to doing that and it is the nursing home's responsibility to sustain life.

I can't express my disbelief right now. I feel we are all finally on the same page now. We are at another road block. We can't take any steps forward to end Dad's daily suffering. I don't know what it will take. God only knows.

Friday, December 21st 2012

My cousin, Karen, came down to visit a friend in Vero Beach. She contacted Mom and planned a visit with Dad. She also brought her therapy dog. Dad enjoyed seeing them both. The following picture is Cousin Karen as a child and Uncle Stanley (Dad's only remaining sibling). Dad enjoyed looking at that picture.

I haven't seen Karen since I was a young child on one of my trips with Dad to his hometown of St. Louis.

Although I was working while she was here, I felt bad that I didn't make the effort to see her. I never really felt that I knew her though. How unfortunate for us both.

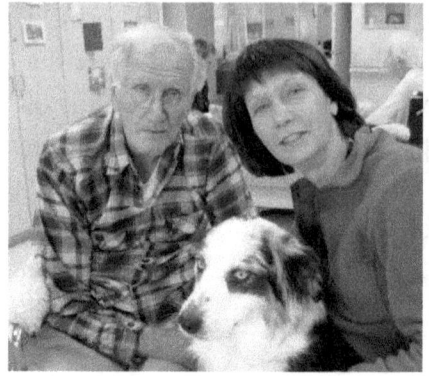 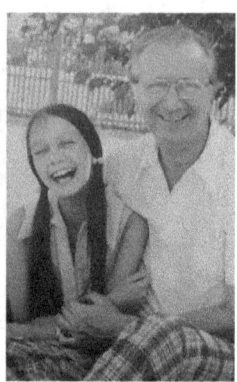

Dad and Cousin Karen   *Karen and Uncle Stanley*

Monday, December 31ˢᵗ 2012

I visited Dad yesterday. Mom and Skippy met me there earlier than usual. Mom said Dad's been very psychotic and difficult the past few days so we thought an earlier visit might work out better. As I approached the entrance into the nursing home, I took a deep breath. I never know how the visit will go or what I'll walk away with. Today, I walked away feeling blessed. As bad as Dad's situation is, there's always someone else who has it worse.

Dad was tearful but happy to see me. When Mom walked away to do something, Dad tried to express his sorrow to me. He locked eyes with me. His eyes showed his thoughts. They pooled with tears. I gave him that moment. Then I told him it would be okay. I gave him a big hug and kiss. He does this often when Mom walks away.

When Mom returned, she told me about Dad's roommate. He was supposed to be there only three weeks or so to receive therapy. It turned out they found cancer throughout him. He sat there stone faced at the other table. I just can't imagine how many hours go by for him in that state.

After speaking with the head nurse, we found that Dad had not been given his 10 a.m. feeding. She said he was quite angry earlier so she held off. Since there weren't many residents in the dining hall, she said she'd come over and give Dad his feeding and medications. Usually, they take the patient to his room to do this. When she came over to us, she was very friendly and sweet with Dad. She was in her early 50's. She had exuberant energy and glowed with beauty. I can only hope to look that good at her age. She told us about all her grandchildren and her dogs. She appeared to be happy in her life. She commented while giving Dad his tube-feeding that a patient can sometimes taste the food in his mouth when it is given. We asked her how she would know that. She openly told us that twelve years ago she was in a car accident and the other driver's pit-bull mauled her face. She had to be tube-fed due to the injuries to her face and body. She was so proud of the work the surgeon did. You couldn't even tell. What a tragic experience. She even shared that she now has a pit-bull as one of her dogs. She said she had to prove to herself that it wasn't the dog's fault. She truly believed that the owners were responsible for raising the dog that way. She said her pit-bull is very sweet. On her phone she showed me pictures of her dog being affectionate toward her. She also shared that her 5 year old dog had recently been diagnosed with cancer. She held herself so strong, so beautiful. I couldn't believe I learned so much about a person I had just met for the first time. I was walking away with such respect for her, for surviving, for living life again.

As we finished our visit with Dad, we started to walk him back to his room. We noticed a little girl running around. She must have been about five. She petted Skippy and made Dad smile. We noticed she was there with some family. They had a cake and it looked like they were going to celebrate something. One of the aides who worked there said to the lady in front of her, "Oh, this is Leonard. I want you to meet him." The lady she was talking to was in a wheelchair. I thought she looked middle age. Her face looked like it had some paralysis. Mom thought she was the little girl's grandmother but the aide said, "She's my sister." She told us she had been in a terrible car accident and almost died. She's been living with the aide (her sister) ever since. They were very kind and Dad said hello in his own way. Again, I couldn't believe what I had just witnessed - the true love and dedication of being there for a family member. The aide works in such a devastating atmosphere - the nursing home. She takes care of sick and dying people. Then she goes home each day to care for her sister. I am without words. I came to visit my father. I came and left with more than I ever imagined. Today's visit pulled me away from my own family's tragedy. It let me see what other people go through. You can't weigh one tragedy as being worse than another. You just have to pray for everyone involved – both the patients and their families.

It's New Year's Eve. I took a deep breath. Three days from now marks a year from when Dad had his stroke. I need to find the strength to help my family, and especially Mom, through this second year. There is no clock on life. A year is a long time. I've learned to take each day as it comes.

"Dad, I'm sorry you have suffered for this long. I blame no one. I've learned blame only prolongs healing. I'll bring you joy in any way I can. I'll be there. I love you, Dad."

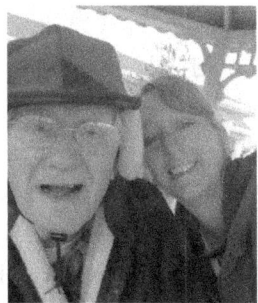

December 31, 2012

Wednesday, January 9th 2013

Mom told me she'd spent the last two days taking care of all the arrangements for when Dad passes. That was such a relief to hear. Mom had been attending some of the Care Giver meetings that were offered through hospice. They strongly recommend that spouses take care of the funeral arrangements before it happens. Waiting will only add more grief to the time of someone's death. I'm proud of Mom for taking another valuable step.

With that, Mom told me about the nursing home drama today. It's such a place of stories. She said she arrived a little early to see Dad today so that she could go to her exercise class right after lunch. She said the nurse caught her coming in and said she was glad she was there. (That's always a concerning comment.) She said Dad was very upset earlier and they've been trying to get him up and out of bed. She said his roommate (the one with cancer) died suddenly and his family hadn't prepared or made any arrangements. So Dad was in there with a dead guy! They said they wanted to get Dad out before the family, or people involved with removing him, showed up. Sure enough, even with the help of an aide, Dad didn't want to get out of bed. We're not sure if he realized his roommate had died or if maybe he was just upset by the commotion in his room. After a while, Mom was able to get him up and out to the patio. She saw people go in, remove the man and drive away in a hearse. By the time Dad returned to the room, it was all cleaned up and empty. I hope Dad didn't understand what had happened to that man. I can't imagine how I'd feel if I were Dad. Such a sobering experience to witness and have to wonder who is going to go next.

After what happened today, Mom was relieved she had made all the necessary arrangements for Dad when it's his turn. We all feel better knowing that Dad won't be waiting on us to be laid to rest. He's been waiting long enough.

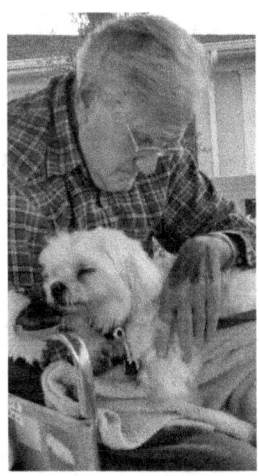

Dad snoozing with Skippy.

Thursday, January 17th 2013

This has been a difficult week for Mom on her trips to the nursing home. Only a day or two went by before Dad got a new roommate. We thought the last roommate was bad - this one topped the scale. Unfortunately, they are all like Dad until they are sedated with heavy prescription drugs. I think Mom carries tremendous guilt when she can't control the issues of the person next to Dad. It's understandable. This week Mom talked about the idea of bringing Dad home again. I guess she feels powerless knowing that when this roommate dies, another will take his place. Bringing Dad home was a scary thing for us to hear, unless we bring him home to die in peace. No matter how much help we hire, it will ultimately take a toll on Mom. Robin talked to her about working out the situation with the nursing home. That was where the change needed to happen. Bringing Dad home wasn't the answer. The nursing home's policy is that if a roommate is a problem for the other patient in the room, then it's the other patient (Dad) who would be moved out but only if space is available. The problem is Dad can't handle change. Nothing in his room can be rearranged or he goes nutty. One time Mom asked a worker to remove the TV from his console because he never turned it on. Dad had a fit when he saw this happening and so the TV is still there. So case in point, Dad's staying put. Just when we got Dad somewhat stable, they throw a more troublesome roommate into the mix.

The next day was better. Mom told me how Dad's been working with his right hand, the one with paralysis. The last few days he's been trying to open and stretch it a little. Something he never attempted before. He would barely ever let Mom work with it. Today, she said he worked with it for quite some time. He was using a cylinder shaped tool to help open the hand. He then put the tool down in his lap as though he was done. Mom thought he was heading back to his room. He ended up wheeling himself over to another resident who had similar physical disabilities. Dad put the tool in the man's bad hand. Mom couldn't believe it. She called over the in-house doctor and nurses to come look. She was amazed he could make that sort of connection. He was working to help someone else with a similar disability. She told me that was the first thing she's seen from him in the past year that reminded her of why she fell in love with him. What a pull on the heart strings.

Monday, January 21st 2013

I had the day off from work today so I went to visit Dad. Mom met me there. I got a good dose of how awful his new roommate is. He is a small, frail old man with eyes the size of saucers. You can't even look him in the eye because his glare is haunting. His voice is loud and strong. Something you wouldn't expect from the looks of him. We found both Dad and his roommate hadn't had their meds yet. What a bad combination. Dad was agitated so I tried to distract him with pictures on my phone while we waited for the nurse to come in. She finally came and got started with his feeding and meds. All the while, his roommate kept shouting for the nurse. He knew she was in the room. He would yell, "Nurse! Nurse!" Then he'd holler, "Where would I be most comfortable?" And the nurse would reply, "Right where you are." This went on for some time. Then he shouted, "Can't you give me something to quiet me up?" followed by "Shut-up!" The nurse looked stunned. She clarified to him that she hadn't said anything. Then he shouted back, "I know. I was talking to myself!" It was hard to watch how Alzheimer's/dementia takes over the mind to the point where a person can't stand to be in his own body.

Through all that commotion, the nurse was telling us about her son. She had adopted a 17-month-old baby from Haiti. He was now in the 4th grade and making strides. She was so proud to talk about him and the struggles she went through to rescue him. It's hard to believe someone in her profession has the energy and drive to take on something like that. She's just another hero among us. When she was finished with Dad, we quickly got Dad up and out of the room and out to the patio. I now see how Mom suffers for Dad. Knowing that he has to share a room with this man, he's now fallen victim to someone else's illness on top of his own.

Wednesday, January 23rd 2013

Tonight I watched the evening news like I always do. They told a story about an older couple. They were making light of how love plays such an extreme role in the recovery of a stroke. The wife had an active lifestyle and career until she suffered her stroke. They showed a clip on how the husband would take her for coffee every day and practice her letter sounds with homemade flashcards in the café. One of the workers who witnessed this daily decided to film a small clip of it on his phone. He posted it on the internet and it got raving reviews. That's probably why it made it to the evening news. Her husband stood by her every day. He would take her to the gym to help regain some of the strength she lost from the paralysis. She spoke slowly in the video and shared her love and devotion to him. She expressed how she couldn't have gotten as far as she had without him. It was touching. I had to hold back the tears as I finished doing the dinner dishes. I felt a range of emotions come over me. For a moment, I felt warm and happy inside, probably like every other American who was watching. What a touching and inspirational story. Then, I thought of Mom and our situation. I felt angry, jealous, disheartened. Look how she pours her love into caring for Dad each day. She spends hours with him. Her day revolves around him. Where is the reward? I don't see it in this year-long picture. But I do believe Dad gets some benefit from her visits. Just a small "something" that reminds him of who he is and the life he once had. She's one of the few people who can retell his story to him. She was there. She remembers.

Unfortunately, the stories Mom tells Dad are so quickly erased from his memory. As for the couple on the news, I can only conclude that it's a fairytale ending to a sad story. It's certainly not our story. I can only wish for a peaceful ending.

Monday, January 28th 2013

Mom called me to say that Dad had another episode. (I call it that because we really don't know what's going on.) He was fine until lunch and then began showing symptoms of a problem. They weren't sure if he was having a stomach blockage or another stroke. They wanted to take him to the hospital but Mom said no. I left work and went to see what was going on. They were sending over a technician to take some chest and stomach x-rays along with taking blood and urine samples. Mom explained to me that if they found anything, it would be a diagnosis that would make him eligible (hopefully) for hospice. Mom was on track about not letting them implement any other life-saving measures. They can treat him for common illnesses but that's all. I still don't agree with all these tests but there are moral and ethical issues that require the nursing home to care and treat him. I agree with that to a point.

A young man entered the room. He said he was there to draw blood. Mom told him that he looked like a teenager. He looked up and thanked her. He said he was 33-years-old and shared with us that he'd been in the Marine Corps. Mom asked him where he served. He said Afghanistan. Mom replied something to the effect that he looked great. He thanked Mom and mentioned he has a metal rod holding his spine in place. He told us he was hit by a road-side bomb. Mom and I stared at each other in disbelief. She asked if they treated him nicely after his service. He said they most definitely did. He said he was awarded two purple hearts and a medal of valor.

I think everyone who walks through those doors is a hero. They just keep showing up.

So once they were done poking Dad, he seemed to be somewhat stable. I said goodbye to him and he tried hard to open his eyes for me. It was that difficult. I thought today that I should have had my poem "Be Free" with me, but I didn't. I'll keep it in my purse from now on. I just don't know when I'll need it.

Tuesday, February 5th 2013

The last week or so has been quite eventful. "Eventful" is never a good word to use in a memoir like this. That previous episode was now making some sense. Dad suffered his first UTI (urinary tract infection) since his stroke. They believe that is what caused the infection last week. So they treated him with antibiotics. During that whole ordeal, his health declined rapidly. Mom wanted to give him time to see if his body would respond to the antibiotics. Just when we thought he was making progress, he showed a new symptom - blood in the urine. So after more tests and x-rays, we still didn't know exactly what was going on. This morning he started passing blood clots. They wanted to send him to the hospital to run more detailed tests but Mom stood her ground, knowing we don't want Dad to go through any more medical procedures. Exploratory surgery is not what we wanted him to go through. I believe that was a good decision. Many people don't understand that he can't comprehend much language other than simple commands or questions. So when a doctor wants to move him to a hospital, do x-rays, or run tests, they don't realize how much fear he has because he doesn't understand. It's just too cruel to make him go through that. They were able to put in a catheter at the nursing home to help drain the clots. It's not a cure by any means but it's what we believe was acceptable treatment at the time.

We never thought this stage of life would be such a fight. We've been fighting for nature or God (whichever it is) to lead the way. I feel Mom has given her heart, her soul, given up everything, to give Dad the best circumstances and environment to live out his last days. She's an incredible person - another hero.

I visited Dad today before the staff meeting. He was out on the patio with Mom. He seemed comfortable and alert. He laughed with me and told me everything that's been going on. I listened intently but couldn't make sense of any of his words. I'll never let him know that though. Mom handed me some papers she had prepared for the meeting. Dad quickly snapped them up with his good hand. He looked them over as if he was reading them; just the way he use to read the morning paper. Mom was anxious. She thought he still might be able to read. The hope is still there.

It's amazing to watch two people grow old together, but then see one who becomes so weak while the other bears all the strength. Mom has shown me that it's not about fairness, being just, or past faults. It's just how you show love in the end.

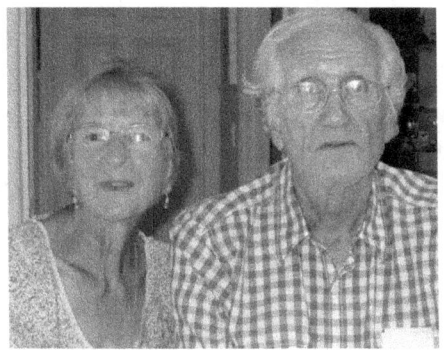

Mom and Dad

Wednesday, February 13th 2013

Well, Dad has overcome this last health crisis on his own. Just last week I didn't think he'd recover. All my life, I was taught to take care of my family and friends. To most of us, it's human nature to act that way. That's where the guilt comes from. Deciding against sending him to the hospital was a terrible feeling to bear, yet I knew it was the right decision for Dad. I've learned you have to be unbelievably strong to push away more chances for life.

They removed Dad's catheter and his plumbing returned to normal without surgery. The bleeding and clots cleared up on its own. I often underestimate the strength and resiliency of the human body. Dad is back to his old happy/grumpy self and the family . . . we're just trying to keep up.

Sometimes I feel overwhelming emotion about this whole journey. Other times it's quite numbing. I'm sometimes amazed when I don't cry or get upset. I worry more when I'm like that because I think I unconsciously put up a wall. But the wall is not made of brick. It always falls. I try so hard to notice how much good I do have in my life. I just wish Dad could see, understand and live it with me while he's here.

Last week I picked up a paintbrush to paint a landscape scene. I was making it to use as a sample for the Art Club that I was going to start teaching. It's been a long time since I've painted. It felt like magic. My hand knew just what colors to dip the brush in and blend it on the canvas. I haven't felt that free in a long time. I think I'm starting to experience a little bit of that blessing of being the art teacher this year. It's a connection with my inner self that seems to be finally coming back.

Sunday, February 17th 2013

Mom called me on Friday to tell me that the nursing home had been quarantined. An intestinal virus was on the loose and there was a lock down at least until Monday. I felt bad for Dad. He doesn't understand what's going on. Even worse, he doesn't understand why Mom isn't coming to visit. Just when you think a situation is stable, life throws something like this in the mix. Robin and Justine were going to come down and visit for the three day weekend, but they canceled. It made no sense since they couldn't visit Dad anyway. Mom is coming down to my house today. Hopefully she will enjoy the break from it all. I just have to hope that Dad is okay. It's an awful feeling when you know there is nothing you can do to comfort him through this.

Monday, February 18th 2013

Mom and I went to a meeting with the attorney who has been working on Dad's guardianship. Mom was focused and confident with her documentation of all the IRA's, several banks, withdrawals and all the other necessary paperwork. I was overwhelmed by the whole business end of this. I couldn't believe the amount of time, money and effort that goes into making a budget for Dad. Everything has to be accounted for and submitted to the judge. I can't imagine if I ever have to take over one day. I'm scared to death because it's possible it will happen. The attorney then made an unnerving comment. She said, "Now that we have a budget for this year, preparing for the next year will be much easier." My stomach sank. I just took a deep breath.

Sunday, March 3rd 2013

It's been three weeks since I've seen Dad. Last week he ended up getting the stomach virus that was running rampant around the nursing home. He survived that. I couldn't risk visiting him while that was going on. That's like running toward a fire rather than away from it.

I finally got the chance to visit Dad yesterday. Mom met me there. Dad was happy, but tearful to see me. Soon after he composed himself, we got him up and out of bed. Then in walked Robin. It started all over again. It was another tearful reunion for him and for her. Then Mom and I just cried along with them. It's a contagious sadness.

The rest of the visit went well. We had lunch with Dad. We do most of the eating. Then we strolled down the hall to the ice cream parlor.

Mom has been telling me all of the attempts she's made lately to get Dad to enjoy an ice cream cone. She would tell me how he would keep turning them down and she'd end up eating them. I thought to myself, "If you're Dad and you can't even enjoy a cup of ice cream anymore, what's left?"

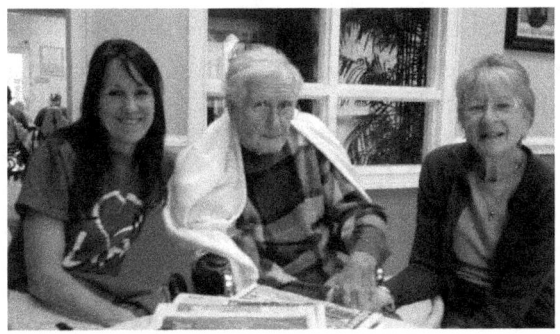

Robin, Dad and Mom in the ice cream parlor.

Not sure what came over Dad that day but he ended up eating some ice cream with us all. I think he did it more for us than for himself.

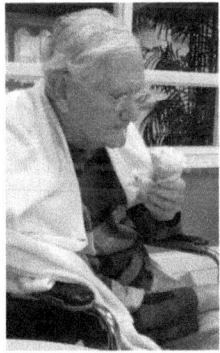

Dad eating his strawberry ice cream.

Mom told us that the horrible roommate wasn't coming back. We weren't sure where he went but there aren't many options at that point in your life. It's usually the hospital or hospice. Mom has been much more at ease since he's been gone. I guess you'd call that a blessing. On our way out, I heard an elderly patient yelling to another that she had to leave. She said she had a mom, dad, brothers and sisters at home. It was obvious her parents were no longer alive. Yet, in her world, they were.

Dad accompanied us to the door and watched us leave through the small window. We all had another bout of sadness as we walked away. Robin and Mom were able to turn and wave to Dad through the small window. I couldn't.

Chapter 6

ARE THE LITTLE THINGS ENOUGH?

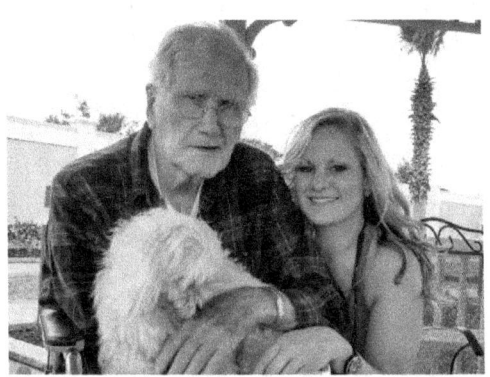

Dad and his oldest grandchild, Justine.
March 25th, 2013

Saturday, March 23rd 2013

It was nice to see Justine with Dad during her visit. She has really grown-up to be a caring person with a big heart. Her sincerity during her time with Dad and her stay with Mom was up-lifting. She fixed Mom's TV and went through pictures and old DVD's Dad had made of the family. It really showed her dedication to her family and especially her grandpa. It was a memorable moment for me. I was able to see something special come out of this unfortunate situation.

Saturday, April 6th 2013

This was a unique and pleasurable weekend. Lori and Robin both came to visit. Robin's husband, David, came too. Mom, Lori and I all have birthdays within the same week. We had a nice visit with Dad for a "pretend" lunch and then we went and had ice cream. Dad took his meds that day so he was cooperative and pleasant. He hasn't gotten a new roommate since the last one left. That has helped tremendously, especially for Mom. Afterwards, we went back to Mom's house and my husband, Dave, and the boys joined us for a dinner celebration. It's been a long time since we've done something like that.

Mom's going to an eye specialist next week to see about scheduling a procedure to remove the cataracts and correct the astigmatism. She says it's been blurring her vision. We reassured her that we would take off work and do the driving to help her and to visit Dad. She says that Dad expects her every day, so she feels an obligation to go. I understand that. It saddens me to know she feels so tied to Dad's care on a daily basis. But it's just how it is. I'm glad I can be there for her since he can't in so many ways.

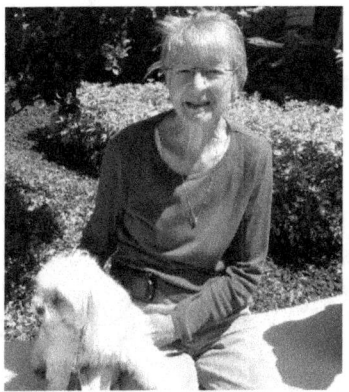

Mom and Skippy

Saturday, April 13th 2013

I had a nice visit with Mom and Dad today. Often Mom says it's not necessary for me to come and that I should enjoy time with my family. She says Dad is okay and not to worry. I don't know if she realizes that my visits to see Dad are also to see her. I need to know she's okay. It's such a monotonous routine she tackles each day.

As I met Mom at the nursing home, she was out on the patio, as usual, tending to Dad. She is always doing something … cutting his hair, applying lotion to his skin, filing nails, whatever he will allow her to do. It's interesting, yet annoying, to see how particular Dad is about which foot to lotion first, which sock to put on, which shoe. It really captures a glimpse of his personality and how it still exists through it all.

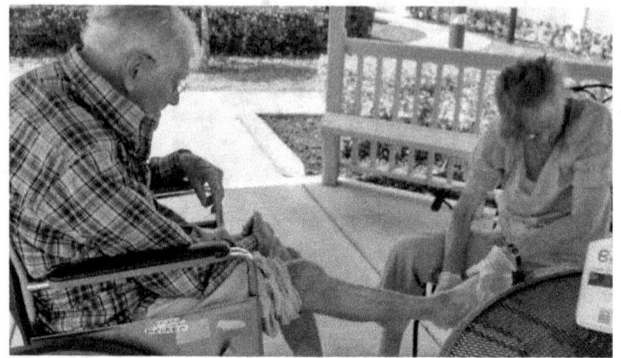

Mom applying lotion to Dad's feet.

As Mom went into the building to get something, I pulled out a watercolor set and set it up for Dad. I was pleasantly surprised how he took to it. I guided him like I guide my young art students - hand over hand, verbally discussing the colors and strokes. When Mom came back out she was thrilled to see this. She always tells me I'm such a good therapist.

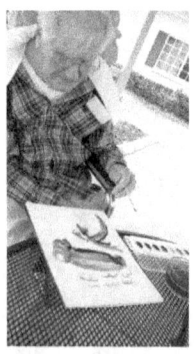

Dad painting with water colors.

Visits have typically been good lately. I almost feel that Dad is okay to some degree; that he has somehow accepted this place as where he must live and understands when we leave. He seems to be able to enjoy most of our visits. I also wonder if I'm just so used to the situation that I've buried much of the pain I feel for him.

We had our "pretend" lunch outside and went for ice cream. It was a little crowded at the ice cream parlor so we were inching our way through. One man, a visitor, was in the hallway. There were two people in wheelchairs, a man and a woman. He began to move the one occupied by the woman out of our way. He turned back to the man in the wheelchair and casually stated, "I'll be back for you Dad." I glanced up at Mom in disbelief. Mom said she's seen this situation before, where both parents are patients. I can't even begin to contemplate the kinds of emotions such an ordeal would entail. It was another reminder that no matter how bad things may seem, there's always someone else suffering alongside you and many times in a worse way.

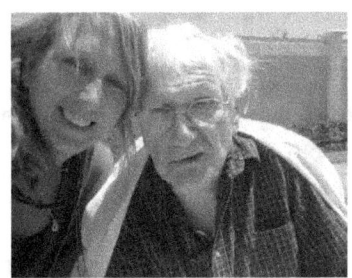

Aimi and Dad in the courtyard.

Saturday, May 11th 2013

I went on my traditional Saturday visit to see Dad today. As we sat outside, I played him a recording of the song, "Raindrops Keep Falling on My Head." We both sang along. He truly enjoyed the experience of knowing the song and being able to mouth and sing some of the words. It was more than Mom could take. Her eyes watered up as she watched. I held strong and kept singing. When Mom went inside to get Dad a drink, he showed me some sadness in his eyes and in the way he held my hand. I haven't seen that for a while. When I went to say goodbye to him at his doorway that's at the end of the hall, he was adamant that he escort me out. He wheeled himself all the way to the exit door and watched me leave through the tiny window in the door. Then he blew me a kiss. It was just heartbreaking.

Mom is preparing for her eye surgery next week and will stay with me for a few days. I don't want to think about how long her vision has been an issue for her. Usually Mom has to be in pretty bad shape to go to this length to fix it. I know she also is doing this because of the responsibility she has toward caring for Dad. She can't afford to fall apart. Putting this burden on her children is not what she wants. I just hope we can keep up with her health as time goes on.

Sunday, June 2nd 2013

Mom stayed with me a few nights while she had her eye surgery. Everything went well and now she is back at home. She wasn't able to visit Dad one of those days. The following day when she went to see him, she found he had written her phone number on a napkin. It was posted in his room. To know he took the initiative to write it as best he could and try to get someone to call for him is … so sad.

For the last few visits Mom got Dad on a project of planting flowers in pots out in the courtyard. It seems to bring him joy each visit as he shows me the blooms and new buds. It gives him a small level of responsibility to water them and check on them each day. During Robin's visit I played Dad the song, "Send in the Clowns." She was massaging Dad's back and I was holding his hand as he tried to sing the words. No sooner did I look up and Robin had tears dripping down her face. Within moments, we were all crying. It's such a beautiful song. Music seems to bring out our weakest emotions.

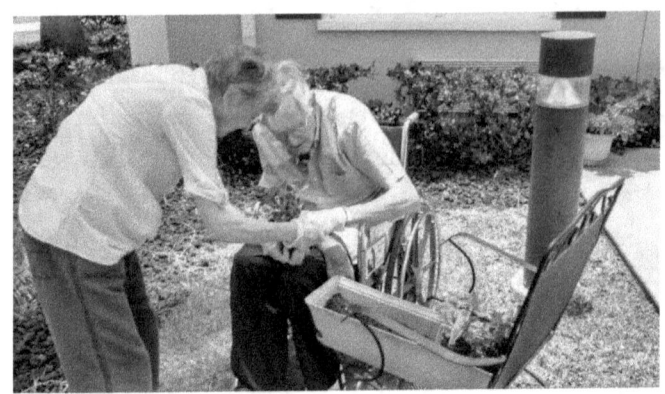

Mom and Dad potting plants.

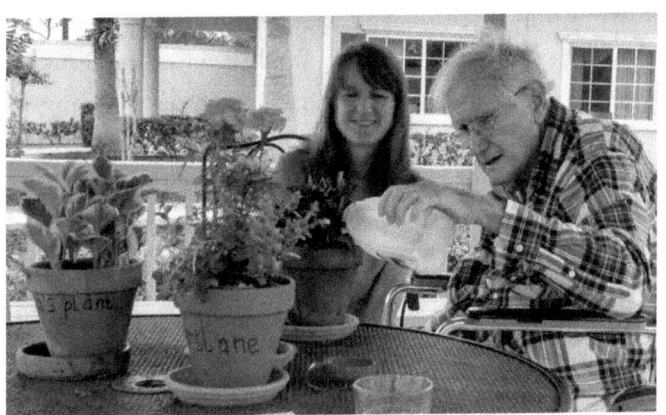

Robin and Dad watering flowers.

On my drive home, my mind started putting together another poem.

Is it Enough?

Is it enough to have to wait for a family member,
To take you outside for some fresh air?

Is it enough to water and nurture a plant,
With the summer heat approaching?

Is it enough to try and mouth the words of a song,
That's still somewhere deep within you?

Is it enough to see someone's life through pictures,
When you can no longer be there?

How do you measure "enough?"
And when do you know when "enough" is still worth living for?

Aimi Medina - June 2nd, 2013

Chapter 7

MORE SPECIAL DAYS, MORE INNER STRENGTH

Wednesday, June 12th 2013

I knew it wouldn't be long before we'd have to go through some tough days again. But here we are. Dad just had his 83rd birthday and Father's Day is this Sunday. I wasn't able to make it on Dad's birthday but Mom told me about it. She said Uncle Stanley sent Dad a birthday card. On Mom's next visit, she handed it to him. He started crying before Mom told him anything about the card. Dad had recognized the handwriting and knew just whom it was from.

Picking out a Father's Day card wasn't easy this year. When your father's mental and physical condition has changed so drastically, most cards are not appropriate, especially the funny ones I used to get him. I managed to find one but it's not the Father's Day card I would have picked a few years ago. It won't be the conditions that I wanted to see Dad live through on Father's Day either. The bottom line is, he's still my dad, and he's still with us, no matter his condition.

I went to visit Dad today. Mom met me there. Since she goes every day to see him, people stop and say hello to her. I never really paid attention to all the "Moms" that are around. There are so many wives, like Mom, who do just what she does. They come every day with a bag in their hand. They try and see if they can get their husbands out of bed and down to the main room. The women look beautifully put together. They smile, they're friendly, and they're just like Mom. They suffer the same burden as she. Their health is declining as well. Some are in their second marriage and don't have anyone there to help support them. They all worry like Mom. They all wonder if they will outlive their husbands and fear what may happen if they don't.

The crape myrtle trees are in bloom in the courtyard at the nursing home. This is the second summer I've seen them bloom here. I worry about how many more summers there will be. I think I'll plant one in my yard when I can no longer enjoy them with Dad.

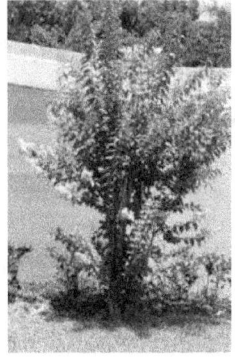

Crape myrtle tree in bloom.

Sunday, June 16th 2013

Today is Father's Day. The parking lot was crowded. I gave Dad his card and read it to him. I glued pictures of all his kids and wrote our names next to them. Mom fell apart as I read the card. I almost did, but I needed to be the strong one, I guess. We had a nice visit. As we were leaving, the lady at the front desk commented that Mom always wears the most beautiful blouses. I agreed. It made me think about all the "Moms" who come to visit and how most of their husbands don't have the words or thoughts to tell them just how beautiful they are. I think I'll make that a point to tell them each time I see them.

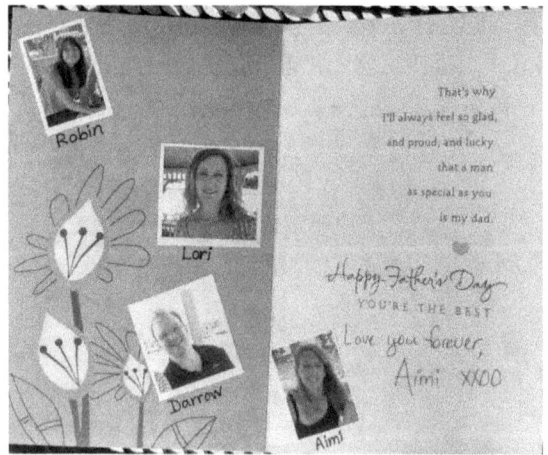

Dad's Father's Day card.

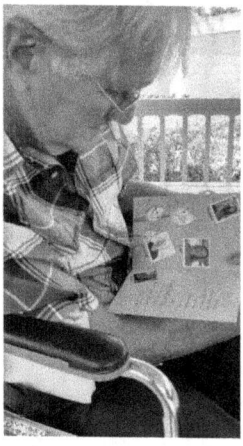

Dad reading his Father's Day card.

Sunday, June 30th 2013

Mom recently came upon her 51st wedding anniversary. I won't use the word "celebrated" because that word just doesn't sound right to use. She made Dad a simple card to acknowledge this day. I can only imagine how difficult that was for her. All I can think about are the wedding vows that I spoke on my wedding day. "For better or for worse, in sickness and in health, until death do us part." Those words only hold true for some.

We had a quiet visit today. Mom brought Skippy and we sat out on the patio. Dad noticed a mockingbird singing and made a motion that he enjoyed listening to it. It was more beautiful than any song I could ever play for him. Once the storm clouds gathered and became threatening, Dad made another motion to go inside. He showed a little authority in this decision. It was nice to see him making a decision and looking out for us. He was being my Dad.

We went inside and Dad nibbled a few bites of his lunch. Then we strolled over to the free ice cream parlor that opens daily at 2 p.m. I got Dad a strawberry cone that he shared with Mom. Mom says now he won't eat ice cream unless she shares it with him. I think it's those little moments, a small connection of love that keeps Mom going.

Over these past few weeks, I've decided to share my story. Not now. I don't know when or with whom at this time. Even if it's only for me, it will be worth it. I've realized these are the most heart-felt words I've ever written. These pages go beyond any art work I've ever done.

This past week my family and I went on vacation to Big Pine Key. When the boys would go off fishing, I started the editing process. I really haven't gone back and read too much of what I've written before this. I found it extremely hard. I was taken aback by the emotion I felt and the things I shared. The mind so easily forgets. Sometimes that's a good thing, but it's also important to remember the hurdles I've been able to live through. The healing will take time, but I'm amazed how strong I've become because of it. I guess Dad will decide the ending of my story and when that will be.

Wednesday, July 10th 2013

Time 3:33 p.m.

Thursday, July 11th 2013

I'm not sure exactly why I looked up to see the time yesterday but sometimes I think it's important to look for signs. Although, I'm returning to this journal page to add my feelings about why I documented the time, I just happened to look up again at my phone clock. It read 2:22 p.m. - that's a little weird.

Saturday, July 13th 2013

If I ever feel the desire to publish this memoir, I've been thinking of some possible titles. I think the title may have a lot to do with how and when this story ends.

Monday, July 15th 2013

Dad has had a nice break lately by not having a roommate. We knew it would only be a matter of time before another one moved in. Sure enough, the facility called Mom to tell her he was getting one. I've seen the roommate a few times since then, and he's been pretty quiet. I asked Mom what she thought of him. She said something to the effect of him being wonderful. I've never heard anything positive come from Mom about Dad's past roommates, mainly because there wasn't anything good to say about them. She said he's been calm and pleasant. She believes he's dying of kidney failure. Everyone in there has something they are dying from. He goes by the name of Bill. He used to write poetry and keeps some in his drawer. He's allowed Mom to read them. She said he wrote beautifully, but it sadly portrayed his life as an alcoholic. I hope to be able read some on a future visit.

It's interesting to learn about the people who stay there. Many were professionals and had amazing talents. That's what's sad about watching Dad interact with others at the facility. No one there knew Dad the way he was before his stroke. That's not to say he was the most liked person in the room, but he was my Dad. All the people and staff who know him now, think he's sweet when he blows them kisses for helping him. However, they also understand the other side of him and have learned to leave him alone when he's agitated. That's about all they'll ever know.

I've been thinking about my nephew Davy's wedding that is planned for early November. His fiancée, Chelsea, and he plan to be married in Georgia. I haven't asked Mom if she's going. I don't think she will, due to the distance and time away from Dad. I had a dream last night. I dreamed Mom was real sick at the house and Lori and I were going to leave her to go to the wedding. It was a horrible feeling. I felt like I was leaving a child behind, knowing that she couldn't safely care for herself. Waking up, I realized I would never have left Mom like that. My dream gave me a clear understanding of how Mom feels about leaving Dad. I don't think she can or will leave Dad for anything. Sadly, I can understand why.

Tuesday, July 16th 2013

During Mom's phone call yesterday, she told me how she took Dad out to get ice cream. Patients who are in the "Nourishment" section have Alzheimer's/dementia, or some other significant diagnosis. They cannot access the rest of the facility unless someone takes them out. Dad's been mostly cooperative lately. He's allowed Mom to take him out and bring him back in without a fight. As they were eating ice cream, she noticed Dad was eyeing the double doors outside the ice cream parlor. Those doors are the exit from the facility. Mom said she was worried Dad was getting an idea in his head to leave. She heard some music from the nearby cafeteria so she distracted him by heading over there. A man was playing the guitar and people were gathered around. She said Dad was mouthing the words to the song and enjoying the music. After the song was over, the people began to clap. Dad can't clap due to the paralysis in his right arm. So Mom used her hand against Dad's and they clapped together.

Thursday, July 25th 2013

I went to visit Dad today. We had a pleasant visit and I got to hear more about Dad's roommate, Bill. Mom said the other day Bill saw her with a CD cassette player that she uses to play music for Dad. He told her he had some cassettes in his drawer of him singing. He asked if she would play some for him. Mom was packing up to leave at the time and told him she would set it up for him the next day.

The next day, Mom asked Bill if he wanted her to set him up in the dining hall so everyone could hear. He declined and told her it had been a long time since he sang. So Mom wheeled him and Dad just outside their room. She set up a table and the music player. When the music played, Bill began singing. Mom was astounded by his voice. She said it was so beautiful. Dad sat across from him and encouraged him to mouth and sing the words. (That's what Dad would do when he worked as a speech therapist with stroke patients.) I asked Mom if anyone ever comes to visit Bill. She said, "rarely." Sometimes people come from his church but not often. Mom said the other day they were praying by his bedside. She said she got upset by this because that usually happens when they know the person is dying. They apologized for upsetting Mom.

I saw Mom interacting with Bill today. She had saved the newspaper for him. When she gave it to him, he told her that he has trouble with his eyes and he didn't have his glasses. I asked Mom why he didn't have glasses. She told me that his doctor checked his eyesight and it was perfect. So, in his mind, he can't read without them. If someone would just get him a pair of clear lenses, if someone was just there, they would know this. I think Mom unknowingly has taken him under her wing. It must be hard to see him every day without someone by his side. It's all too common there. Mom is spread so thin, yet, she's there for him too - unbelievable.

Chapter 8

THE LAST CHAPTER

Wednesday, July 31st 2013

I received a call from Lori that afternoon and she was panicked. She said the nursing home had called her because they couldn't get in touch with Mom. They said Dad was sick and coughing up phlegm. They wanted to send him to the hospital for tests. Lori was adamant that they not send him for more testing. We told them early on that we would not put Dad through any more procedures; only those they could do at the nursing home. We decided that I would go directly to Mom's and pick her up. That way she wouldn't have to drive herself. (It turned out Mom missed the call because she was vacuuming.)

When I arrived, Mom was in her swimming pool doing her exercises. I walked around the back of her house to the screen door of the pool. She was surprised to see me twice in one day, especially since I didn't call. I told her she needed to get dressed and that Dad wasn't doing well. She didn't panic. She calmly got out of the pool and went in to get dressed. This was the start of our next crisis.

When we arrived, the nurse briefed us. She said the doctor wanted to send Dad to the hospital for x-rays and blood work. Mom said no but agreed they could do those procedures there at the facility as they had in the past.

As we waited around, Dad's roommate, Bill, shared with me his poetry. It was beautiful and sad like Mom expressed. It's amazing how something so devastating as alcoholism could be so understood and brought to light in his writing. He also gave me a CD of him singing. I told him I would listen to it and return it the next day. He insisted that I keep it but I also know how quickly one can forget.

Just before 11 p.m. the x-ray technician arrived. He was able to get a stomach x-ray and noticed something concerning. He thought maybe Dad had had a previous surgery. When we said he hadn't, he apologized for any worry. The doctor would be able to explain the results. So, as far as we knew, still no one had come to draw blood and the doctor wouldn't see the x-ray until morning. We decided to leave. I would stay at Mom's house in case we had to return in the night. On our way out, a daughter of one of the patients was also leaving. She said the other day she arrived after hours and had to go through the night entrance. When you ring the doorbell at the night entrance an employee will let you in. However, she said no one came. Dad saw her and kept trying to wave down a staff member to help her. She told us how he's so sweet and blows her kisses. It felt good to hear that.

Thursday, August 1st 2013

My backup had arrived. Both Lori and Robin came to help. Dad was getting agitated because he hadn't had any of his medicines since the previous morning. The nurse tried to give Dad a feeding with his meds. She only got a small cup of water with a Tylenol down before she stopped suddenly. We could hear a gurgling in his throat. After reporting this to the doctor, a chest x-ray was ordered. The doctor thought maybe Dad had aspirated. All food and water had now been stopped until the doctor could determine what was wrong. Words cannot express the inner pain I'm feeling for Dad right now.

Friday, August 2nd 2013

Early this morning, Mom and I showed up. Dad was in a bad way. (I'll just leave it at that.) Finally, we were able to meet with the doctor. He said the blood results showed Dad was in renal failure, his chest x-ray was okay which meant he didn't aspirate. This was the turning point. The nursing home doctor explained that Dad was suffering from an upper small intestinal blockage. The doctor then explained our options. He told us there was nothing else he could do at the facility to clear the blockage. He also didn't think that Dad was a good candidate for surgery. He believed that Dad might not survive the operation. He then asked us which direction we wanted to take. I had no idea today would bring us to this decision. We asked if he would now agree to bring in hospice. He willingly supported our decision and set up a meeting with hospice the next day. I felt somewhat relieved knowing Dad's suffering would finally come to an end. Little did I realize just how painful it would be.

Saturday, August 3rd 2013

We made our makeshift office in the hallway just outside Dad's room. We quietly took chairs from the adjacent rooms and rolled out Dad's table as a desk. Many times I wanted to step out the glass double doors next to Dad's room to get a breath of fresh air. Then I would remember you need a code to open them. It's a reminder of how Dad must feel sometimes. Once we were set up, we just hoped none of the nearby residents would go into one of their delusional rages or put on what I call a "Broadway Show." We were getting use to camping in the hallway.

A little later the hospice counselor arrived. We went through the standard admitting questions. We had most of it in place due to our prior visit back in December of 2012. We told her our request was to have hospice come to Dad. He was still very aware and at ease with the staff that cared for him. She said the hospice nurse would meet with us that same afternoon and go over any details with us.

The time couldn't have moved more slowly. All we wanted was for them to give Dad something to relax and get rid of the pain. We finally met with the hospice nurse who was ready to take charge. She was going to have things in place to start morphine drops by that evening, or so we thought.

Sunday, August 4th 2013

On my early drive to see Dad, I popped in the CD that Bill had given me to listen to. His voice took me back in time. I was serenaded with him singing Sinatra songs like "Old New York" and "Georgia." It's amazing to hear how talented he was and that people had come to listen to him. As I drove I sadly thought, "Where are his fans now? He's at the end of his journey alone." Next thing I knew, I was there. I took a deep breath.

When I entered Dad's unit, I was in disbelief. Dad was dressed, in his chair and wheeling around in the dining room where they were serving breakfast. Mom and Robin had just walked into this situation and were bewildered as well. It turned out that they had only just started the morphine 4 hours earlier. This was one of the worst things I've had to witness. Dad was looking for his tray. He even wheeled over to the aide who was passing out small juice containers to residents watching the morning church service on the big TV. We did what we could to lure Dad back down the hallway to his room. He then tried to get into Mom's lunch cooler. Something he's never shown interest in. We quickly got the nurse to come over and give him his next dose of morphine for which he was long overdue. He was becoming agitated. Once the nurse approached him, we knew this would be a battle. Dad wouldn't cooperate and it wasn't long before all of us got involved in helping to restrain him. Robin kept telling him it was okay, while Lori tried to hold his good arm back. The nurse was busy trying to get the medicine in, while I was pulling Mom back from trying to help. Once we were finally successful, Dad calmed down. Robin appeared to hold herself together after this. The rest of us just cried like babies. We were all sick to our stomach.

After the storm, the cleaning aide who had witnessed the whole event told us she'd been working there for years and had never seen a more dedicated family as ours. And I thought we were just standard. To top it off, Dad's roommate, Bill, had to tell me how great Dad looked. I thanked him and handed him his music. He was glad he was able to share it with me. He says he doesn't sing much anymore because the words don't come to him like they use to. He appreciated that I returned it. It was sad to see the deceptions within his world. They are all too common here.

From then on, we were in charge. We took turns guarding Dad's door. We made sure he didn't leave and that he had his medicine on time. Mom sent me home because she had Robin to stay with her to help monitor Dad.

As I lay in bed that night, I thought about the poem I had hoped to read to Dad today. I still couldn't bring myself to do it. I glanced at my phone clock I was holding. It read 11:11 p.m. I can only interpret these times as signals of a countdown. That would only make sense.

Monday, August 5th 2013

Lori went back home to Miami. She would return in a few days and bring her boys. I met Robin and Mom at the nursing home this morning. One of the nurses on a new shift wasn't up-to-date on Dad's status. She thought she would resume feedings because a certain amount of time had passed since the doctor put a "Hold" on his chart. We nearly fell over. She even thought that we could try giving him honey. She obviously had not been briefed on his care. She missed the big sticker on his folder that said he was under hospice care. We may seem like the worst people in the world by stopping all food and water but it's what needed to happen. Up to now, this nursing home provided him with the care he needed. But they weren't equipped with what he needed for death. We wanted him to leave this world with dignity. We knew what we had to do.

This had been a horrific day so far. One dose of morphine was given past the time that Dad had needed it. Because of this, he became combative and Robin had to help restrain him to get it in his mouth. Everything after that was just bad. He was agitated and still in pain. He wouldn't let us touch him. He would kick and show amazing strength as he lashed around uncomfortably in his bed. I don't know how to describe what it felt like to see Dad this way. Pain like this can't even be shown in tears.

Later that morning, we were able to meet with the hospice nurse who was able to adjust Dad's medications to be given sooner and more frequently if needed. We discussed our new decision to move Dad to the hospice house. She was glad to see we reconsidered and understood why.

That afternoon, the hospice physician came to visit. He checked Dad out and went over all his charts, recent tests and x-rays. He said that with all Dad had going on, he was surprised he was still alive. He said most people in his condition would have died days earlier. He agreed to have Dad moved to the hospice house and would send a critical-care nurse to stay with him until the move took place. We agreed to the plan but they wouldn't be able to coordinate the move that late in the day. It would have to be tomorrow. So we agreed to bring in the critical-care nurse for the time being. The only drawback was that some facilities like this one won't allow other nurses to administer medications. So she could only make sure that the nurses on shift gave it to him when they were supposed to. We were okay with that. We really couldn't do anything more.

Now it was late afternoon. All this time I had my "Be Free" poem in my back pocket. No one else was in the room at the moment so I pulled it out to read it to Dad. As I tried to read the first line, Dad pushed me away. At this point, he wouldn't accept a comforting hand any more. Had I missed my chance? Heartbroken, I put it away and told Dad to be free, to let go. Before I left, I told him goodbye. I touched him in the gentlest way and he pulled away. I told him I loved him and I would be back soon. He gave me a slight nod with his head. His eyes remained closed and his body tight and curled.

Finally, the critical-care nurse showed up and said she would make sure Dad got his medication before the agitation and pain was uncomfortable for him. We were all beyond exhausted. We went home to get some rest. We knew tomorrow wouldn't be easy.

I left around 6 p.m. I cried the whole way home. I was angry. I was furious. I just didn't know exactly at whom. Dad was going to fight to the very end. It was beyond sad, it was beyond ugly. It was devastating. I don't know if I'll see him alive tomorrow. I'm scared of what tomorrow will bring. I don't want him to die this way.

Tuesday, August 6th 2013

Day 5: No food or water. How is this possible and why won't he let go? The critical-care nurse was there when we arrived that morning. We were glad he had someone to stay with him through the night. He was still fighting us against giving him any meds. It was so hard to see him that way.

Finally, things were in line to move Dad to the hospice house. Around 2 p.m. the van came. Of course at the same time we were trying to move Dad out, there was a 911 call for someone else in the unit. It was a chaotic exit but at least it happened.

We arrived at the hospice house that was only a mile away. They were very attentive to Dad's needs and got him comfortable. The doctor came in to see him. He said his pulse was still quite strong. Once again, he was amazed at Dad's will to fight.

Once Dad was settled, Robin and I went back to the nursing home to collect Dad's belongings. We gathered up all the pictures and his nice shirts. We left many things knowing that soon they would be of no use to him or us. It was hard to leave his shoes behind. We said goodbye to many of the people and residents that had been so kind to Dad. We said goodbye to Bill. I felt bad leaving him alone to finish his journey. Even Dad's buddy, Ed, whom he often sat with at lunch, came in his room looking for him. We told him we were moving Dad to another place. I think he knew. Many people in passing would remind us how Dad would blow them kisses. This was not easy to hear. I knew we wouldn't be back.

We then returned to the hospice house. Dad was unaware of what was going on but he looked at ease. Robin and Mom decided to head home. I stayed to say goodbye. Mom insisted that I go home and get some rest. I said I would. I just wanted to stay a little longer. I finally had another chance to read my poem to Dad. As I read him the poem, he showed no emotion or response. That was okay. I know he heard me. I left it folded in his hand. I was hoping I could be there and help him let go. That didn't happen. That was okay too. I wanted him to do it his way, with or without me. I then walked away and headed home. At least he had my poem with him now. He had heard my words.

Robin and Mom returned later that evening and found my poem in Dad's hand. I apologized if it upset them but I wanted Dad to have it with him. They understood. Robin said they were due for a good cry anyway. Mom spent the night with Dad thinking he'd pass in the night.

Wednesday, August 7th 2013

Day 6: No food or water for six days, an upper bowel obstruction, renal failure, an infection, gurgling in the throat. How is this possible?

I went over to see Dad just before 8:00 a.m. I thought maybe I'd have one more chance to see him or maybe have the chance to be with him when he passed. Surely, it would be this morning, although I know there aren't any rules to this chapter.

The wonderful nurses came in to give Dad a sponge bath. Mom and I didn't think he'd live through that. Well he did. They have been keeping him medicated and comfortable. Comfortable is an interesting word because I hadn't realized or remembered what Dad looked like in a comfortable state. For 19 months, I haven't seen his body relaxed as it was today. I haven't seen his facial muscles smooth and without tension. As I was relieved to see him this way, I also had to witness Dad dying. His eyes were no longer a way for him to speak. His body had used every fat calorie that was gained from being over-fed from all the formula. His cheek bones were pronounced as his body was just taking and taking. His breathing had changed with slow pauses in between. I never wanted to see my dad die. I never thought how strong I'd have to be so that he wouldn't have to.

We spoke to the doctor again. He said Dad could pass at any time but he could also hold on for one to two more days. I just couldn't believe he just spoke those words.

I sat outside with Robin on the beautiful porch entrance. We talked about Dad and our disbelief in his survival. What is he waiting for? We have reassured him on all levels. I have held his hand and gave him the choice to die with me at his side. We have given him the choice to die alone or with Mom or Robin. I have written him my most precious words in poetry. I have sung to him. I have played his favorite songs. I have given everything I can think of.

As I sat at his bedside, I watched his chest rise and fall - hoping it was his last breath. How cruel is that to say? It's not, if you truly love someone and know it's time for God to take over.

A little later that day a volunteer from hospice was visiting our room and talking with Mom. Mom told me she allowed her to read the poem that I wrote for Dad. It was still folded in his hand as he rested. She told me it was beautiful and brought tears to her eyes. She asked if I have ever published anything. I told her I hadn't. She said she use to write down the most heartbreaking stories of her visits to Haiti. She'd write about the devastation and lack of care they have there. How she would try and care for the sick and dying babies that all had diarrhea and worms. There were no supplies and the rains kept the diapers from drying. She told me she wrote her experiences down for herself. It was not intended to be shared. I told her it takes courage to share your writing. She agreed. She said it makes you vulnerable and shows your inner self to the world. She also said that if it can help even one person, then it's worth it. She finally found the courage and is about to publish her book. Knowing that Dad had been silent for 19 months, she said I should write down my story. She said being there is what can help others. I looked up at her and told her that I have written it all down and it's called, "Being There." Her facial expression was that of surprise. It felt that she knew things before I told her. This is another one of those people I speak of as heroes. I somehow felt that I was supposed to meet her today. She didn't even know me and she was giving me the courage I needed. I've only told one person, my son Jonny, that I was writing a book. I only told him because he's very observant, and I believe those are the little steps to gaining confidence.

Just last night, I wrote something to read at the funeral when it's time. Ironically, it said just what I discussed with the hospice volunteer today. It reads, "For the last 19 months, Dad has had to stay silent throughout this entire journey. I have been writing a memoir called, *Being There* where I have let my heart speak out for him through my words and tears. I have experienced heartbreak, learned lessons, met heroes, and learned to appreciate something so difficult and yet so beautiful, we call *life*. I want to thank you, Dad, for giving me the strength to tell your story. I hope to one day have the courage to share it. I can now write the last chapter and we can end this journey together as a family."

I didn't tell my family sooner about me writing a book because I didn't want it to change or filter any feelings or conversations that I felt were so important in keeping this story true. It was meant for the purpose to allow me to heal. You can't do that when you're writing from your heart and someone is judging you. That's why it was necessary to stay silent, just like Dad.

Four-thirty in the afternoon came around and Dad was still with us. Mom was making her plan for the evening. Robin would take her home for a while and bring her back for the night. I couldn't believe that I would have to leave again with Dad still holding on.

I drove home wondering if this would be the last time. Yesterday, I left angry. Today, I left frustrated. We have suffered alongside Dad for this long. He's so close. But on this day, he wasn't ready. I have to remember it's his story. He writes the ending.

As I was nearing the expressway exit, I realized I didn't have anything to wear to Dad's funeral. I know Mom doesn't want a black somber gathering. Blue has always been Dad's favorite color. I ran into a nearby store and grabbed every blue dress. I felt myself talking with Dad in the dressing room, somehow giving him the choice. I found one and headed home. I usually enjoy shopping. This task brought me no joy. I do wonder if I'll ever wear this dress again. It will either bring me happiness or it will hang quietly in my closet as just a memory.

Chapter 9

SAYING GOODBYE

Thursday, August 8th 2013

Today was the day. I just didn't know it yet. Darrow had flown in at one o'clock in the morning. Robin insisted that he see Dad at hospice. There was nothing else we could think of that would be keeping Dad holding on, other than saying goodbye to Darrow. Was this what Dad was waiting for? Was he waiting for his son? So Darrow paid his respects to Dad during his visit. Mom spent the night again with Dad at the hospice house and Darrow and Robin went back to Mom's house to sleep.

I woke up this morning in disbelief. No one called. I knew what that meant.

I rushed this morning. This was now my standard routine: down two cups of coffee, pack survival food, emergency stay-over bag, text Robin, and out the door. This was one more opportunity to be there. Maybe he did want me at his side. My heart ached knowing that he suffered another night.

I was there about seven in the morning. Mom was sleeping in a pull-out bed. She woke suddenly when I entered and wasn't sure what was going on. I jokingly said

I was a guardian angel and that confused her more. I reassured her that everything was okay and nothing had changed with Dad. She was so exhausted she actually fell back asleep. I pulled a chair up next to Dad and told him I was there. I held his hand but I knew even his hand was losing a connection with me. Dad had a wet wash cloth over his forehead. His eyes were glossed over. I knew the only thing left was his sense of hearing.

A little later, Robin had arrived. She walked in quietly and heard me singing to Dad. She asked me what the song was. I told her it was "Rainbow Connection," a song that I loved as a child. Dad and I loved the Muppet's. It was one of the classic songs from the movie. My old childhood friend and I used to sing it together. We still have a lifelong connection. Later in life, I sang it to my own children when they were young and I would put them to bed. And now I was singing it to my Dad.

A little while later, Darrow arrived and Mom was up. The nurse came in. She looked Dad over and then showed us his feet. They were blotchy in color. She told us this was part of the process. His blood supply was now staying in his core to work his vital organs. She also told us that she would no longer turn Dad as they had been doing. Every so often they would rotate Dad from laying on one side and roll him to the other for comfort and circulation. I knew the time was near.

I made sure Dad's poem was in his hand. I reminded him about what it said. After holding Dad's hand for some time, I noticed an odor. It was on my hands and it wasn't pleasant. I went over to the sink and washed them with soap. After holding Dad's hand again, the odor returned. Was this the smell of death? I cringed to even think about it. I couldn't connect with this. I've never experienced this before so I wasn't sure how to understand it. I washed my hands again and moved forward. I knew that sound was more dominant than touch, so I focused on talking to him. It's what I had to do.

After taking turns being at Dad's side, Robin and Mom went to the kitchen to eat their breakfast. I decided to stay next to Dad. I watched him. I watched his breathing. It was changing. The nurse warned us he might take a deep breath and then start again about ten seconds later. Before long, I started to see it happen in front of me. I didn't know what to do. I didn't want to leave his side but I wanted Robin and Mom to be there. Darrow was there but he had a bad back so I knew he wouldn't move fast enough to get them. I decided to text Robin and hope she would get it. At 11:06 a.m., I texted her with one word, "Come." Soon, she and Mom ran in the door. I didn't have to explain. They understood. We gathered around Dad and reassured him that it was okay. We told him we loved him. Then, he stopped breathing. We each questioned each other as to whether he was still with us or not. By 11:14 a.m., we pronounced his death.

We cried with sorrow and relief. Robin and I finally had the hug we'd been waiting for. The hug we never thought would happen. It was the hug that finally meant that Dad was at peace. After a good cry and a family melt down, it was over. It was finally over.

After our goodbyes, it quickly became an awkward situation. The nurses came in. They had called the funeral home and a few men entered the room. This is where I had to believe that Dad was no longer in his physical body. I had to believe that his spirit was now above us. As they had Dad ready to take away on a gurney, we all began to walk away. I found myself running back and asked the men if they had Dad's poem. They said they did and that it was in his hand. I asked them to keep it with him and they reassured me they would. I then walked away for the last time.

That day, the rest of the family drove to Mom's. They were all ready to come days before but we kept telling them to wait because Dad wasn't ready. We then planned a simple ceremony with just the family.

As I lay awake that night, I thought about those numbers that I saw on my phone clock a few weeks back. They had read 3:33 p.m., then the next day 2:22 p.m. I made my own interpretation that something I couldn't explain was giving me a countdown. On the day Dad died, I looked back to see what time I had sent the text to Robin and Mom to "Come." It read 11:06 a.m. We pronounced his death at 11:14 a.m. Somewhere in between the tears and saying goodbye, that clock read 11:11a.m. Looking back at the calendar, he died exactly 30 days from the day I noticed the 3:33 p.m. time. I can't explain it, but I feel in my heart, I was right. I just think someone greater knew it before me.

Friday, August 9th 2013

Today, we buried Dad. Mom had asked everyone to share a memory of Dad at the ceremony, even the grandchildren. This was the first time in a long time we had the chance to think of Dad in a positive light. Everyone had something to contribute. The grandchildren spoke first. Justine talked about Dad's love for National Geographic, photography and the old movies they would watch together. Davy remembered his fascination with dinosaurs and how Dad would share books and fossils with him. Austin shared how Dad would give him unlimited ice cream at his house. Kyle talked about the time they bought a blow-up whale for the pool from CVS pharmacy that was already inflated. He had to hold it in the open convertible all the way back to the house. Noah remembered going to the Strawberry Festival with Dad and winning lots of prizes. Drew loved how Dad would put a bag over his head when he would visit and pretend he was the Boogie Man. Jonny retold his memory of the thousands of CDs Dad owned and how he would sit in Dad's comfortable chair listening to music blast through his expensive speakers.

His children then spoke. Robin remembered his compassion for animals (but he always enjoyed a good steak), his love of loud music (but everything else should be quiet) and most of all, the love he had for his family (although he could be hard to love at times.) Lori remembered the Friday nights he would take one child with him to Sears. On her turn, she would walk around the store with him and then get to pick out the Swedish fish or chocolate turtles from the candy counter. Darrow shared how Dad's dedication to our family lives on through all of us. We've all raised our own children with strong morals and beliefs like he had. Darrow had a "move forward" attitude that was strong and positive. I got up and shared a few of my poems. As I started to speak, I froze. Dave came up and stood by my side as I regained my strength to go on. I shared my "Father's Day" and "Be Free" poems. My family knows I always speak from the heart. As difficult as it was to read, I had to look above my son, Drew's, tear-filled eyes. Other family members shared jokes and funny stories about Dad. That's what we needed. That's why we were there.

Lastly, Mom shared some poetry as well. One of which she wrote herself, entitled, "A Poem for Leonard." I found it to be incredibly valuable. The poetry she shared expressed that even in marriage the love between two people can come and go but if you stick with it, it returns. I thought that was an important message for all her children and grandchildren to hear. It validates Mom's commitment to being there for Dad these last 19 months. It goes like this.

Poem for Leonard

When Love is gone,
Love is gone,
Like a ripple on the pond,
Like the perfume in the breeze,
Like the rainbow from the sky,
Like a misty morning sun.
When Love is gone
Love is gone.

When Love returns,
Love returns,
Like a tide of ocean currents,
Like the earth beneath our feet,
Like the bass underwater flashing,
Like petals opening to sunshine.
When Love returns,
Love returns
For ever.

Susannah Becker 2010

Chapter 10

THE LOOKING GLASS

Monday, August 12th 2013

Today was the start of moving forward. I know it will take some time because the wounds are deep. As I reflect on a few things, I say them in the hope that someone will read Dad's story and make some decisions about their own life. I challenge you to think about yourself and your loved ones. What would you want done or not done to you? Whom do you trust to make healthcare decisions in accordance with your wishes if you become unable to make them for yourself? Write it down and make it a legal document. You can tell everyone your wishes until your blue in the face and it won't matter. Death is a tragedy in itself. There is no need to prolong it with pain and suffering because you were given false hope.

Dad's situation was a combination of things. He was not specific in his living will. He didn't specify which life sustaining treatments he would or would not accept. His will was written primarily in the event of his death. He appointed Mom as his health care surrogate but nothing else. She would only have access to any financial accounts in the case of death – as his beneficiary. Only being caretaker allowed her to access his funding for him but only under a judge. That is why Mom had to struggle through the court system to be his legal guardian. The other factor was the feeding tube. The neurologist along with the surgeon should have consulted together, and with us as a family, about our options. That never happened. Due to the massive stroke and Dad's age, it should have been apparent that Dad's chances for a recovery, one that would sustain a quality of life, was minimal. We as a family should have been able to think that decision over and decide for him. We also didn't understand early on how difficult it would be to have the feeding tube removed. The medical professionals always lean toward sustaining life. The fight to remove it was too difficult for Mom to bear. She felt the responsibility of her guardianship weighed more heavily than making decisions as his wife of 51 years. Many times we requested the tube only be used for medications, which would have given Dad the choice to eat or not - a choice many people make on whether they choose to live or die. The request was always denied. We were told that he would starve to death without it. The ironic thing about all this is that that is how he ultimately died. On top of an upper bowel obstruction, renal failure, an infection, and a heart made of steel, he continued to suffer six more days without food or water. There are no words that can be brought to paper to express the heartache of witnessing his last days. Forever, I will hold close to me his love, his strength and the musical rhythm of his heart. It will carry me to my journey's end.

I am proud of Mom for achieving her one goal she set back when Dad suffered his stroke. Her goal was to outlive him. She did it. Thank God. Now we hope she'll find the strength to move forward without him and fill her days with happiness; something she's missed out on for too long. We'll hold her hand until she lets go.

Dad's journey has ended. I can now full-heartedly say that he is no longer suffering. But it took leaving this world for that to happen. He is now at peace; he is free. I can now imagine him listening to his classical music again, enjoying his morning bagels, and looking down on me when I need him. That's how I need to remember him. One thing we as a family made sure of was that he didn't go through this alone. We suffered alongside him. We listened even when there were no words for him to speak. He died knowing he would be missed and was loved by us all. I know this to be true because I made a choice. I was there.

ABOUT THE AUTHOR

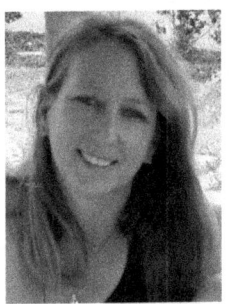

Aimi Medina grew up in Coral Gables, Florida. She has been living in Vero Beach, Florida for the past fifteen years with her husband, Dave, and their two children, Drew and Jonny. She earned a Bachelor of Science degree from Florida International University in elementary education and is a certified teacher with the state of Florida. She later became certified in art. She now teaches art to students at a local elementary school. She continues to find art, in all its forms, a way to express and share the tender moments of life with all who listen.